REFERENCE

DICTIONARY OF

AIDS

RELATED

TERMINOLOGY

...REY T. HUBER, Ph.D.

Neal-Schuman Publishers, Inc.
New York   London

Published by Neal-Schuman Publishers, Inc.
100 Varick Street
New York, NY 10013

Printed and bound in the United States of America

Library of Congress Cataloging-in-Publication Data

Huber, Jeffrey T.
    Dictionary of AIDS-related terminology / edited by Jeffrey T.
Huber.
      p. cm.
    Summary: Includes definitions of over 1000 abbreviations and
acronyms, historical and medical terms, key names, and sources of
information found in discussions of AIDS and HIV.
    ISBN 1-55570-117-5
    1. AIDS (Disease)—Dictionaries—Juvenile literature. [1. AIDS
(Disease)—Dictionaries.]   I. Title.
RC607.A26H895   1992
616.97′92′003—dc20
                                         92-31265
                                            CIP
                                            AC

This book is presented as a tool to help bridge the communication gap within the AIDS arena and is dedicated to all individuals who have been affected by this pandemic.

CONTENTS

PREFACE

The terminology associated with the acquired immunodeficiency syndrome (AIDS) and the human immunodeficiency virus (HIV) is growing rapidly as we learn more and more about AIDS and HIV. In addition to redefining existing terms, the pandemic has created its own vernacular, encompassing many medical, legal, social, psychological, and religious issues. In addition, an increasing number of individuals and organizations are becoming involved in the fight to stop the spread of the virus. As the pandemic continues to grow, the number of words and names associated with it is likely to increase even more.

This *Dictionary of AIDS-Related Terminology* is an alphabetical list and explanation of key words, names, and phrases generally found in discussions of AIDS and HIV. The dictionary includes abbreviations, acronyms, historical terms, key names in the AIDS arena, medical terminology, drugs associated with past and present therapy, major organizations and institutions, and AIDS-specific sources of information. Dates, histories, biographies, addresses, and telephone numbers are included where appropriate and available. Cross references are provided from abbreviations, acronyms, vernacular, and product names to the main entry.

Every attempt has been made to make the definitions herein accessible to the widest possible readership. In cases where key terms have complex medical definitions, these are preceded by shorter, simpler explanations to serve readers who do not require the complete definitions.

Since the acquired immunodeficiency syndrome and the human immunodeficiency virus involve many complex, everchanging issues in a variety of subject areas, this work should not be regarded as a comprehensive listing of every term, person, source of information, or organization. Rather, it is intended as a guide to the most common terminology included in discussions of AIDS and HIV at the time of publication. To get the most current information about drug therapies and other factors that change rapidly, consult an AIDS service provider.

ACKNOWLEDGMENTS

The editor gratefully acknowledges the assistance of Patricia B. Carroll, M.D., Assistant Professor of Medicine and Surgery, University of Pittsburgh, and R. Stephen Almagno, O.F.M., Professor, School of Library and Information Science, University of Pittsburgh, in the compilation of this book. Without their continued support, it would not have come to fruition.

A

AAPHR *see* American Association of Physicians for Human Rights

Abbott Laboratories A pharmaceutical company based in North Chicago, Ill. Among its many other products, Abbott manufactures the antibody test to detect the presence of the human immunodeficiency virus. It also produces numerous educational materials concerning HIV and AIDS. Abbott Laboratories, Abbott Park, IL 60064, (708) 937-6100.

abortion The induced termination of pregnancy. Symptoms commonly experienced during abortions include uterine contractions, uterine hemorrhage (sometimes including tissue), dilation of the cervix, and ejection of fetal material.

abscess A localized collection of pus resulting from the displacement or disintegration of tissue in any part of the body.

ACHA *see* American College Health Association

achlorhydria 1) The absence of hydrochloric acid in the gastric juices. 2) The absence of hydrochloric acid in the stomach secretions, a result of the atrophy (wasting away or diminution in size) of the gastric mucous membrane. *Also called* gastric anacidity.

ACIDS *see* acquired community immune deficiency syndrome

ACLU *see* American Civil Liberties Union

acquired community immune deficiency syndrome (ACIDS) One of a group of names initially used to denote the acquired immunodeficiency syndrome. The current name was adopted in 1981. *See also*

1

community acquired immune deficiency syndrome, gay-related immune deficiency, and acquired immunodefiency syndrome.

acquired immune deficiency syndrome   *see* acquired immunodeficiency syndrome

acquired immunodeficiency syndrome (AIDS)   Illness characterized by infection with the human immunodeficiency virus (HIV) coupled with the presence of one or more of a constellation of opportunistic infections or diseases (such as Pneumocystis carinii pneumonia, Kaposi's sarcoma, and candidiasis) and the absence of any other known cause of immunodeficiency. AIDS does not include all manifestations of HIV-related illnesses. *Also called* acquired immune deficiency syndrome. *See also* AIDS-related complex, human immunodeficiency virus, and person with AIDS.

Note: The Centers for Disease Control and Prevention surveillance case definition is divided into three sections, depending on the laboratory status of HIV infection. When laboratory tests for HIV are not available, and the patient has no other cause of immunodeficiency, the following definitively diagnosed diseases may be construed to indicate AIDS: a) candidiasis of the esophagus, trachea, bronchi, or lungs; b) cryptococcosis, extrapulmonary; c) cryptosporidiosis with diarrhea persisting for more than one month; d) cytomegalovirus disease of an organ other than liver, spleen, or lymph nodes in a patient over one month of age; e) herpes simplex virus infection causing a mucocutaneous ulcer that persists longer than one month; or bronchitis, pneumonitis, or esophagitis for any duration affecting a patient over one month of age; f) Kaposi's sarcoma affecting a patient less than 60 years of age; g) lymphoma of the brain (primary) affecting a patient less than 60 years of age; h) lymphoid interstitial pneumonia and/or pulmonary lymphoid hyperplasia (LIP/PLH complex) affecting a child less than 13 years of age; i) Mycobacterium avium complex or Mycobacterium kansasii disease, disseminated (at a site other than or in addition to lungs, skin, or cervical or hilar lymph nodes); j) Pneumocystis carinii pneumonia; k) progressive multifocal leukoencephalopathy; l) toxoplasmosis of the brain affecting a patient longer than one month.

With laboratory presence of HIV infection, any disease listed above as well as any of the following may indicate AIDS: a) bacterial infections, multiple or recurrent (any combination of at least two within a two-year period), of the following types affecting a child less than 13 years of age: septicemia, pneumonia, meningitis, bone or joint infection, or abscess of an internal organ or body cavity (excluding otitis media or superficial skin or mucosal abscesses), caused by Haemophilus, Streptococcus (including pneumococcus), or other pyogenic bacteria; b) coccidioidomycosis, disseminated (at a site other than or in addition to lungs or cervical or hilar lymph nodes); c) HIV encephalopathy (also called HIV dementia, AIDS dementia, or subacute encephalitis due to HIV); d) histoplasmosis, disseminated (at a site other than or in addition to lungs or cervical or hilar lymph nodes); e) isosporiasis with diarrhea persisting more than one month; f) Kaposi's sarcoma at any age, g) lymphoma of the brain (primary) at any age, h) other non-Hodgkin's lymphoma of B-cell or unknown immunologic phenotype and the following histologic types: small noncleaved lymphoma (either Burkitt or non-Burkitt type) or immunoblastic sarcoma (equivalent to any or the following, although not necessarily all in combination: immunoblastic lymphoma, large-cell lymphoma, diffuse histiocytic lymphoma, diffuse undifferentiated lymphoma, or high-grade lymphoma); i) any mycobacterial disease caused by mycobacteria other than Mycobacterium tuberculosis, disseminated (at a site other than or in addition to lungs, skin, or cervical or hilar lymph nodes); j) disease caused by Mycobacterium tuberculosis, extrapulmonary (involving at least one site outside the lungs, regardless of whether there is concurrent pulmonary involvement); k) Salmonella (nontyphoid) septicemia, recurrent; l) HIV wasting syndrome (emaciation or slim disease). In some cases, the patient's condition will not allow for definitive tests.

Presumptive diagnosis is indicative for AIDS under these circumstances for the following: a) candidiasis of esophagus; b) cytomegalovirus retinitis with loss of vision; c) Kaposi's sarcoma; d) lymphoid interstitial pneumonia and/or pulmonary lymphoid hyperplasia (LIP/PLH complex) affecting a child less than 13 years of age; e) mycobacterial disease (acid-fast bacilli with species not identified by culture), disseminated (involving at least one site other than or in addition to lungs, skin, or cervical or hilar lymph nodes); f) Pneumocystis carinii pneumonia; g) toxoplasmosis of the brain affecting a patient longer than one month.

The Centers for Disease Control and Prevention is expected to amend the surveillance case definition of AIDS in 1993 to include pulmonary tuberculosis, recurrent pneumonia, invasive cervical cancer, and a CD4+ T-lymphocyte count less than 200.

ACT UP   *see* AIDS Coalition To Unleash Power

ACTG   *see* AIDS Clinical Trails Group

active anal intercourse   *see* insertive anal intercourse

acupuncture   A technique developed in China for treating pain or inducing anesthesia by passing needles into specific points of the body. The patient remains conscious throughout the procedure.

acute   1) Sharp, severe, poignant. 2) Having sudden onset with a short and severe course. 3) Not chronic.

acute encephalopathy   1) Any degenerative disease of the brain with a short or relatively severe course. 2) Any reversible deterioration of mental status or cognitive function.

acute HIV exanthem   A severe skin eruption or rash that manifests itself with the human immunodeficiency virus.

acyclovir   1) A drug used to treat herpes and sometimes used as an adjunct to AZT. 2) An antiviral drug that is effective against herpes simplex virus infections, including types 1 and 2, varicella-zoster virus, cytomegalovirus, and Epstein-Barr virus. It is used for infections of the genitals and herpes infections of the skin. The trade name is Zovirax.

ADC   *see* AIDS dementia complex

Addison's disease   A disease resulting from a deficiency or lack of secretion of adrenocortical hormones. It may be a result of tuberculosis-induced or autoimmune-induced disease of the adrenal glands. It is characterized by anorexia, fever, tumors, hemorrhagic necrosis, weight loss, hypotension, weakness, and occasionally a discoloration of the skin. If not treated, it is usually fatal. *See also* adrenal insufficiency.

adenine arabinoside   *see* vidarabine

adenopathy   Swelling or enlargement of the lymph nodes.

adenovirus   One of a group of related viruses that cause disease in the upper respiratory tract. These viruses have also appeared in latent infections in some people. Many types of adenoviruses have been isolated and assigned numbers. In addition to human adenoviruses, there are also various types found in animals.

adolescent   An individual during the period marked by the beginning of puberty until maturity. This period is a gradual process and varies among individuals. It is classified by the National Library of Medicine as ranging from age 13-18, but other institutions and disciplines define it as broadly as ranging from age 11-25.

adrenal function   The action performed by the adrenal gland.

adrenal insufficiency   Abnormally low or decreased production of adrenal corticoid hormone by the adrenal gland. Addison's disease is the result. *See also* Addison's disease.

adult respiratory distress syndrome (ARDS)   1) A form of lung disease in which an abnormally large amount of fluid is present in the tissue. 2) A restrictive lung disease caused by increased permeability of the pulmonary capillaries or the alveolar epithelium. The condition often develops after severe infection, trauma, or systemic illness. It has approximately a 50-percent fatality rate.

Advil   *see* ibuprofen

aerosolized pentamidine   An anti-infective drug produced as a colloidal solution and dispensed as a mist for inhaling. It is effective against Pneumocystis carinii pneumonia.

African Swine Fever   A viral disease caused by an immunologically distinct agent and first isolated in Africa. It has also been found in Brazil, Cuba, the Dominican Republic, Haiti, and western Europe. It was considered early in the epidemic to have possibly been the causative agent of the acquired immunodeficiency syndrome.

agent   Something that causes a biological, chemical, or physical effect. Bacteria that cause a disease are agents of that disease; medicine administered to cure a disease or an illness is a therapeutic agent.

AHA   *see* American Hospital Association

AHG   *see* Factor VIII

AHMA   *see* American Holistic Medical Association

AIDS   *see* acquired immunodeficiency syndrome

AIDS Action Council   Founded in 1982, this organization functions as a representative of AIDS service facilities in Washington, D.C. It lobbies Congress on AIDS-related issues, monitors federally funded research, produces various publications, and maintains a speakers' bureau. AIDS Action Council, 2033 M Street, N.W., Suite 801, Washington, DC 20036, (202) 293-2886.

AIDS Clinical Trials Group (ACTG)   The National Institute of Allergy and Infectious Diseases (NIAID) trial network for AIDS drugs. NIAID contracts with institutions to perform the actual drug trials through a grant process, with a principal investigator controlling the trial. AIDS Clinical Trials Group, National Institutes of Health, 6003 Executive Boulevard, Room 200 P, Rockville, MD 20852, (301) 496-8210.

AIDS Coalition to Unleash Power (ACT UP)   An AIDS activist organization founded in 1987 by Larry Kramer. It was originally formed to fight for the early release of drugs that could be used in the treatment of AIDS and is devoted to increasing public awareness of the epidemic. The organization's motto is "united in anger and committed to direct action to end the AIDS crisis." ACT UP, 496A Hudson Street, Suite G4, New York, NY 10014, (212) 989-1114.

AIDS dementia complex (ADC)   1) A condition in which the human immunodeficiency virus affects the brain. It can result in a loss of mental capacity. 2) A constellation of neurologic symptoms caused by infection with the human immunodeficiency virus and characterized by global impairment of intellectual function. It is usually progressive and interferes with normal social and occupational activities. *Also called* HIV encephalitis, HIV encephalopathy, multifocal giant-cell encephalitis, and subacute encephalitis.

AIDS enteropathy   Any intestinal disease manifesting with the acquired immunodeficiency syndrome. *See also* acquired immunodeficiency syndrome.

AIDS Health Service Program   A program created and implemented by the Robert Wood Johnson Foundation to assist with the high cost of AIDS care and treatment. The program is funded through grants from private foundations and addresses the ways in which health care services are organized. It covers Florida, Georgia, Louisiana, New Jersey, Texas, and Washington. *See also* AIDS Service Demonstration Program, AIDS-specific Medicaid Home and Community-Based Waiver, and Designated AIDS Center Program. AIDS Health Service Program, c/o Robert Wood Johnson Foundation, P.O. Box 2316, Princeton, NJ 08540, (609) 452-8701.

AIDS Knowledge Base   An online database prepared by health care professionals associated with the San Francisco General Hospital, the University of California, and various affiliated institutions that covers all aspects of AIDS. AIDS Knowledge Base is also available as a CD-ROM product and in print. The database is available from BRS Information Technologies, 1200 Route 7, Latham, NY 12110, (800) 345-4277. The print version is published by the Massachusetts Medical Society, Medical Publishing Group, 1440 Main Street, Waltham, MA 02254, (617) 893-3800. The CD-ROM product is part of the Massachusetts Medical Society's COMPACT LIBRARY: AIDS package.

AIDS Medical Foundation (AMF)   A nonprofit organization founded in 1982 by Dr. Mathilde Krim that promoted AIDS research and provided funding for its support. The Foundation merged with the National AIDS Research Foundation to form the American Foundation for AIDS Research in 1985. *See also* American Foundation for AIDS Research.

AIDS.NET   An electronic bulletin board that serves the deaf and hard-of-hearing populations. AIDS.NET, International Deaf/Tek, Inc., Deaftek.USA, P.O. Box 2431, Framingham, MA 01701-0404, (508) 620-1777.

AIDS prodrome   Any sign or symptom indicative of the onset of the acquired immunodeficiency syndrome. *See also* acquired immunodeficiency syndrome.

AIDS Project Los Angeles   One of the early AIDS service organizations founded in the United States. It continues to be the main service provider in the Los Angeles area. AIDS Project Los Angeles, 6721 Romaine Street, Los Angeles, CA 90038, (213) 962-1600.

AIDS-related complex (ARC)   A group of signs and symptoms such as fever, persistent generalized lymphadenopathy (PGL), and weight loss accompanied by the presence of human immunodeficiency virus antibodies. Originally used in cases of HIV-infected individuals not diagnosed with AIDS but with compromised immune systems and decreased T-cell counts, the term is now widely considered to be obsolete. *See also* person with AIDS-related complex.

AIDS-related virus (ARV)   A virus isolated from homosexual men in 1984 in Atlanta, Georgia. It was initially thought to be similar to the human immunodeficiency virus.

AIDS Service Demonstration Program   A program created and implemented by the Health Resources and Services Administration to assist with the high cost of AIDS care and treatment. The program is funded by federal grants and addresses the ways in which health care services are organized. It covers Arizona, Florida, Georgia, Illinois, Louisiana, Massachusetts, New Jersey, New York, Pennsylvania, Puerto Rico, Texas, and Washington. *See also* AIDS Health Services Program, AIDS-specific Medicaid Home and Community-Based Waivers, and Designated AIDS Center Program. AIDS Service Demonstration Program, Health Resources and Services Administration, 5600 Fishers Lane, Rockville, MD 20657, (301) 443-6745.

AIDS service organization (ASO)   An institution or consolidated group operating at the local, state, or national level that provides beneficial services to individuals affected by the human immunodeficiency virus, such as medical services, counseling services, legal assistance, housing assistance, and food banks.

AIDS-specific Medicaid Home and Community-Based Waivers   A program created and implemented by the Health Care Financing Administration to assist with the high cost of AIDS care and treatment. It is funded by state and federal Medicaid money and addresses the ways in which health care services are organized. It covers New Jersey and New Mexico. *See also* AIDS Health Services Program, AIDS Service Demonstration Program, and Designated AIDS Center Program. AIDS-specific Home and Community-Based Waivers, c/o Health Care Financing Administration, Department of Health and Human Services, 200 Independence Avenue, S.W., Washington, DC 20201, (301) 966-3000.

AIDS Task Force for the American College Health Association   This organization attempts to educate college students about AIDS and its dangers. AIDS Task Force for the American College

Health Association, Department of Student Health, Box 378, University of Virginia, Charlottesville, VA 22908, (804) 924-2670. *See also* American College Health Association.

AIDS Treatment Evaluation Units (ATEU)   A network of drug testing sites created by the National Institute of Allergy and Infectious Diseases in 1986. National Institute of Allergy and Infectious Diseases, AIDS Program Office, Building 31, Room 7A49, Bethesda, MD 20892-4200, (301) 496-5893.

AIDS Treatment Registry (ATR)   A directory of New York clinical trials created in 1988 by members of the AIDS Coalition to Unleash Power (ACT UP). The Registry was designed to provide detailed information about trials for people who might want to participate. ATR is now produced by the American Foundation for AIDS Research (AmFAR).

AIDSLINE   A National Library of Medicine (NLM) database that contains citations to AIDS-related literature. The citations are derived from various NLM databases, including CANCERLIT, HEALTH PLANNING AND ADMINISTRATION, and MEDLINE. AIDSLINE is available from the National Library of Medicine, MEDLARS Management Section, 8600 Rockville Pike, Bethesda, MD 20209, (800) 638-8480; BRS Information Technologies, 1200 Route 7, Latham, NY 12110, (800) 345-4277; and DIALOG Information Services, Inc., 3460 Hillview Avenue, Palo Alto, CA 94304, (800) 334-2564.

AIDSpeak   A vernacular created by public health officials, politicians, and AIDS activists that has been used by these groups and others to describe various issues related to the pandemic. Among its characteristics is the use of nonjudgmental language.

AIDSphobia   A phrase coined to denote an unrealistic fear and dread of the acquired immunodeficiency syndrome.

AL 721   An egg-based compound developed to remove cholesterol from cell walls, which was tested in Phase I trials for the treatment of the acquired immunodeficiency syndrome. The majority of the research on AL 721 has been done outside the United States, predominantly at Israel's Weizmann Institute of Science, where it was developed in 1979.

allergic dermatitis   *see* atopic dermatitis

allergic eczema   *see* atopic dermatitis

alopecia   Absence or loss of hair where it is normally present, especially of the head; baldness.

alpha interferon   A drug effective in preventing replication of the human immunodeficiency virus in the laboratory (in vitro). A significant limitation of its use in the living body (in vivo) is the toxic effects the drug has on humans.

altered mental state   A difference in the functional state of the mind as judged by an individual's behavior, appearance, responsiveness to stimuli of all kinds, speech, memory, and judgment.

alveoli   Plural of alveolus.

alveolar proteinosis   *see* pulmonary alveolar proteinosis

alveolus   1) A general term used to denote a small, saclike cavity. 2) An air cell of the lung. 3) An erosion or ulcer of the gastric mucous membrane. 4) The socket of a tooth.

AMA   *see* American Medical Association

ambulatory care   Treatment provided to mobile (not hospitalized) patients.

Amcil   *see* ampicillin

ameba (also amoeba)   1) A one-celled, microscopic organism that may infect humans, causing amebiasis. 2) A tiny, one-celled, protozoan organism that inhabits soil and water. It sends out fingerlike projections of protoplasm (pseudopodia) that enable it to move about and through which it obtains nourishment. The pseudopodia also keep the shape of the ameba in constant flux. Amebae reproduce by binary fission, with the nucleus dividing by mitosis.

amebae (also amoebae)   Plural of ameba (amoeba).

amebiasis (also amoebiasis)   The state of being infected with amebae, especially Entamoeba histolytica. Many patients remain asymptomatic. Those who manifest symptoms generally suffer from dysentery accompanied by diarrhea, nausea, vomiting, and weakness.

amebic dysentery   Infection with entamoeba histolytica. *See also* amebiasis.

America Responds to AIDS   An AIDS education campaign launched in 1988 by the Centers for Disease Control and Prevention to promote public awareness.

American Association of Blood Banks   A cooperative organization founded in 1947 consisting of administrators, blood banks, nurses, physicians, transfusion services, and other persons and organizations interested in blood banking. It operates a clearinghouse for blood and blood products, conducts educational programs, trains and certifies blood bank personnel, sponsors workshops, maintains a file on rare donors, and inspects and accredits blood banks. American Association of Blood Banks, 1117 North 9th Street, Suite 600, Arlington, VA 22209, (703) 528-8200.

American Association of Kidney Patients   An organization made up of persons on hemodialysis and peritoneal dialysis, persons with kidney transplants, their friends and families, and professionals in the field. The Association was established in 1969 and works to educate the public about kidney disease, to fight for quality health care, and to promote kidney donations. American Association of Kidney Patients, 1 Davis Boulevard, Suite LL7, Tampa, FL 33606, (813) 251-0725.

American Association of Physicians for Human Rights (AAPHR)   An organization made up of physicians and medical students who seek to eliminate discrimination based on affectual or sexual orientation in the health professions. The Association educates the public about homosexual health care needs and promotes unprejudiced care for gay and lesbian clients. It was founded in 1979. American Association of Physicians for Human Rights, 2940 16th Street, Suite 105, San Francisco, CA 94103, (415) 255-4547.

American Cancer Society   An organization made up of volunteers who support research and education in cancer detection, diagnosis, prevention, and treatment. Special services are provided to cancer patients. It was founded in 1913. American Cancer Society, 1599 Clifton Road, N.E., Atlanta, GA 30329, (404) 320-3333.

American Civil Liberties Union (ACLU)   An association that fights for the rights of people established in the Bill of Rights of the United States Constitution by providing advocacy, education, and litigation services. It was established in 1920. American Civil Liberties Union, 132 W. 43rd Street, New York, NY 10036, (212) 944-9800.

American College Health Association (ACHA)   An organization consisting of institutions and individuals that is concerned with the promotion of health to college students and members of the college community. The Association provides continuing education and seminars for health professionals. It was founded in 1920. American College Health Association, 1300 Piccard Drive, Suite 200, Rockville, MD 20850, (301) 963-1100. *See also* AIDS Task Force for the American College Health Association.

American Foundation for AIDS Research (AmFAR)   An organization dedicated to promoting AIDS research and providing funding for its support. It was founded in 1985 by the merger of the AIDS Medical Foundation and the National AIDS Research Foundation. American Foundation for AIDS Research, 5900 Wilshire Boulevard, 2nd Floor, E. Satellite, Los Angeles, CA 90036, (213) 857-5900.

American Holistic Medical Association (AHMA)   Founded in 1978, it comprises licensed medical doctors, doctors of osteopathy, and medical or osteopathic students who are interested in promoting holistic health care (the integration of emotional, mental, physical, and spiritual concerns with the environment). The Association provides referrals to the public, maintains various committees, and produces several publications. American Holistic Medical Association, 2002 Eastlake Avenue E, Seattle, WA 98102, (206) 322-6842.

American Hospital Association (AHA)   Founded in 1898, this organization comprises health care institutions and individuals concerned with the provision of health services. It conducts research on various aspects of the provision of health care and provides educational programs for health care personnel. American Hospital Association, 840 N. Lake Shore Drive, Chicago, IL 60611, (312) 280-6000.

American Medical Association (AMA)   An organization made up of physicians and county medical societies. Founded in 1847 to disseminate information to its members and the public at large, the Association assists in establishing standards for continuing education, hospitals, medical schools, and residency programs. It lobbies Congress on behalf of its members concerning issues affecting the delivery of health care. The AMA also operates a library and produces various publications. American Medical Association, 515 N. State Street, Chicago, IL 60610, (312) 645-4818.

American Public Health Association (APHA) A professional organization consisting of health care professionals and interested consumers. Founded in 1872 to seek to ensure the promotion and protection of environmental, mental, and physical health, the Association produces various publications. American Public Health Association, 1015 15th Street, N.W., Washington, DC 20005, (202) 789-5600.

American Red Cross An organization founded in 1881 that provides services to members of the armed forces, veterans, and their families; assists in disasters in the U.S. and abroad; operates regional blood centers; trains volunteers; provides community services, including HIV/AIDS education programs; and publishes service-related materials. American Red Cross offices exist throughout the United States. The main office is located at 17th and D Streets, N.W., Washington, DC 20006, (202) 737-8300.

Americans for a Sound AIDS Policy (ASAP) Founded in 1987, this organization advocates a compassionate, enlightened, ethical public policy on HIV and AIDS. It seeks to educate people in order to help stop the spread of HIV, promotes early detection of infection, operates a speakers' bureau, houses an on-site collection of newspaper articles, disseminates information, and testifies to government agencies on AIDS-related issues. Americans for a Sound AIDS Policy, P.O. Box 17433, Washington, DC 20041, (703) 471-7350.

AMF *see* AIDS Medical Foundation

AmFAR *see* American Foundation for AIDS Research

amino acid 1) Any of a large group of organic acids that link together to form the proteins necessary for life. 2) One of a large group of organic compounds containing both an amino group and a carboxyl group. They have the ability to act as both an acid and a base and exhibit properties associated with both the amino and carboxyl groups. They serve as the building blocks for the construction of proteins and are the end result of protein hydrolysis or digestion. Approximately 80 amino acids have been isolated in nature, 20 of which are essential for human growth and metabolism. *See also* amino acid therapy.

amino acid therapy   A questionable form of AIDS therapy available outside the United States, especially in Mexico. The results have not been proven to be long-term.

amniotic fluid   The transparent, almost colorless liquid contained in the inner membrane (amnion) that holds the suspended fetus. It protects the fetus from physical impact, insulates against temperature variations, and prevents the fetus from adhering to the amnion and the amnion from adhering to the fetus. The amniotic fluid is continually absorbed and replenished.

amoeba   *see* ameba

amoebiasis   *see* amebiasis

amoxicillin   1) A semisynthetic penicillin. 2) A semisynthetic derivative of ampicillin. It is effective against a broad spectrum of gram-positive and gram-negative bacteria and is administered orally. Trade names include Amoxil, Polymox, Robamox, and Trimox.

Amoxil   *see* amoxicillin

amphotericin B   1) An antibiotic agent used in the treatment of severe fungal infections. 2) An antifungal antibiotic derived from a strain of Streptomyces nodosus. It is administered parenterally (brought into the body by any means other than the digestive tract, such as intravenous injection) in the treatment of such deep-seated mycotic infections as systemic candidiasis, aspergillosis, cryptococcosis, and histoplasmosis. The drug may also be applied to the skin topically in the treatment of candidiasis and related infections.

ampicillin   A semi-synthetic penicillin which appears as a white, crystalline powder. When administered orally, this antibiotic is effective against various gram-negative and gram-positive bacteria. Predominantly used in the treatment of urinary system and urinary tract infections, it is also used to treat prolonged bronchial infections. Trade names include Amcil, Omnipen, Polycillin, and Principen.

Ampligen   An interferon-inducing drug developed by DuPont that has received limited testing for the treatment of the acquired immunodeficiency syndrome.

amyl nitrite inhalant   A highly flammable and volatile clear liquid that causes blood vessels to relax (or dilate) when inhaled. True amyl nitrite generally requires a prescription, unlike butyl nitrite. It is used recreationally. *Also called* rush and poppers.

ANAC   *see* Association of Nurses in AIDS Care

anal intercourse   Sexual intercourse by insertion of the penis into the anus. *Also called* anal sex. *See also* insertive anal intercourse and receptive anal intercourse.

anal sex   *see* anal intercourse

anal squamous-cell carcinoma   A form of carcinoma located on the anus that develops from the flat, scaly, epithelial cells of the epidermis (those cells that form the outer surface of the body and line the internal surfaces).

anal wart   1) A small tumorous growth, caused by a virus, located on the anus. 2) A circumscribed cutaneous lesion located on the anus. It is caused by a human papillomavirus and is transmitted by contact.

analgesic   1) Relieving pain. 2) An agent that alleviates pain.

Ancobon   *see* flucytosine

anemia   1) A condition in which there is a reduction in the number or volume of red blood cells. 2) A sign of various diseases characterized by a deficiency in the oxygen-carrying material of the blood, measured in unit volume concentrations of hemoglobin, red blood cell volume, and red blood cell number.

anergy   A reduced response to several specific antigens.

angular cheilitis   *see* perleche

angular cheilosis   *see* perleche

angular stomatis   *see* perleche

anilinctus   *see* anilingus

anilingus   Sexual activity in which the mouth and tongue are used to stimulate the anus. *Also called* anilinctus and rimming.

anorectal disease   A pathological condition of the anus and rectum, or the area joining the two, which is manifested by a characteristic set of clinical signs and symptoms.

anorexia   The lack or loss of appetite for food. This is common in the onset of fevers and systemic illnesses, psychiatric illnesses, depression, malaise, and in pathological conditions of the alimentary tract, especially the stomach.

anthrax   An acute, bacterial, infectious disease caused by Bacillus anthracis. It generally attacks cattle, goats, horses, or sheep, but may be passed on to humans through contact with infected animals, their discharges, or contaminated animal products. Failure to properly treat anthrax may be fatal. *Also called* charbon, milzbrand, and splenic fever.

antibody   1) A substance in the blood produced in response to the presence of an antigen to form the basis for immunity. Antibodies generally defend the body against invading disease agents, but the HIV antibody does not. 2) A protein substance, comprised of immunoglobulin molecules with a specific amino acid sequence, developed in response to the presence of an antigen. The antibody interacts only with the antigen that caused its creation, or with those that are closely related. This relationship between antigen and antibody forms the basis for humoral immunity. The presence of antibodies may be linked to vaccination, previous infection, perinatal transfer of bodily fluids between mother and fetus, or unknown exposure. The body also possesses natural antibodies that react without apparent contact with a specific antigen.

antibody testing   The procedure used to determine the presence of an antibody. Testing for the HIV antibody is used to determine if a person has been infected with the human immunodeficiency virus. *See also* antibody.

anticonvulsant   1) Any agent that prevents or relieves convulsions. 2) Preventing or relieving convulsions.

antidepressant   An agent that prevents, cures, relieves, or alleviates depression. *See also* depression.

antidiuretic hormone   *see* vasopressin

antifungal   Any agent that kills fungi, inhibits the growth or reproduction of fungi, or is used to treat fungal infections.

antigen   Any substance that, under specific conditions, has the ability to induce a particular immune response and to react with the product of that response. The antigen induces the synthesis of an antibody. It is this interaction that forms the basis for immunity.

antihemophilic factor A   *see* Factor VIII

antihemophilic globulin   *see* Factor VIII

antimoniotungstate   A drug found to be poisonous to the blood when tested for treating infection with the human immunodeficiency virus. This drug was developed in the 1970s as a potential treatment for Creutzfeld-Jacob disease. It inhibits the reverse transcriptase and has been tested in Phase I and II trials for treatment of infection with the human immunodeficiency virus. It has exhibited hematologic toxicity consistently in these tests.

antineoplastic   1) An agent that prevents the development, growth, or spread of malignant cells. 2) Preventing the development, growth, or spread of malignant cells.

antiviral   Any substance that destroys a virus or inhibits its replication.

antiviral drug therapy   The administration of an agent that destroys a virus or inhibits its replication.

anus   The terminal orifice of the digestive tract, which serves as an outlet for the rectum, located in the fold between the buttocks. *Also called* asshole (slang).

APHA   *see* American Public Health Association

aphtha   A small ulcer on a mucous membrane of the mouth.

aphthae   Plural of aphtha.

aphthous   Pertaining to, or characterized by, aphthae.

apoplexy   *see* cerebrovascular accident

ara-A   *see* vidarabine

ARC   *see* AIDS-related complex

ARDS   *see* adult respiratory distress syndrome

arenavirus   1) A group of RNA viruses that cause a variety of diseases in humans. 2) Any of a group of viruses consisting of multi-shaped virions that have four large and one to three small segments of single-stranded RNA. The presence of ribosomes gives the virions a sandy appearance. The principal virus in this group is the lymphocytic choriomeningitis virus (LCM virus). Also included are the American hemorrhagic fever viruses and the Lassa fever virus. Rodents typically serve as hosts for the viruses.

Armstrong, Donald   Born in 1931 in Montclair, N.J., Dr. Armstrong holds a staff appointment at Memorial Sloan-Kettering Cancer Center, 1275 York Avenue, New York, NY 10021, (212) 639-7809. He is credited with aerosolizing pentamidine in 1986, allowing for direct penetration in the lungs for the treatment of Pneumocystis carinii pneumonia.

arthralgia   Pain in a joint.

artificial insemination   The mechanical injection of semen, which is capable of fertilization, into the vagina.

ARV   *see* AIDS-related virus

ASAP   *see* Americans for a Sound AIDS Policy

Ascomycetes   1) The sac fungi. 2) The largest class of Eumycetes, the true fungi. They are characterized by a sac that encloses the spores. Included in this group are yeasts, mildews, blue molds, and truffles.

aseptic meningitis   The common name for a mild form of meningitis. Most cases are caused by viruses. *See also* meningitis.

ASO   *see* AIDS service organization

aspergillomycosis   *see* aspergillosis

aspergillosis   1) A fungal infection. 2) Infection caused by Aspergillus and characterized by granulomatous lesions in the tissues or on any mucous surface. Areas commonly affected include the skin, lungs, aural canal, nasal sinuses, urethra, and occasionally in the bones or meninges. *Also called* aspergillomycosis.

Aspergillus   A genus of fungi in the family Moniliaceae. After sexual development, it is classed with the Ascomycetes. This genus includes several species of molds, some of which are opportunistic pathogens.

Association of Nurses in AIDS Care (ANAC)   Founded in 1987, this organization consists of nurses and health care professionals involved in the care of persons with AIDS. It serves as a network for its members, provides support services, promotes public awareness and education regarding AIDS issues, and advocates the rights of those infected with the human immunodeficiency virus. Association of Nurses in AIDS Care, 10141 Liberty Road, Randalltown, MD 21131, (301) 922-1446.

asthma   1) A condition in which periodically recurring sudden attacks of difficulty in breathing are accompanied by coughing and wheezing. 2) A condition characterized by paroxysmal shortness of breath accompanied by wheezing caused by spasmodic contractions of the bronchi or bronchial tubes or by swelling of the bronchial mucous membrane. Asthma may coexist with other allergies or may be caused by an allergic reaction. Secondary factors influence the recurrence and severity of attacks such as physical fatigue, mental or emotional stress, and pollutant irritants.

ASTRA Pharmaceutical Products, Inc.   The Swedish-based company that owns the drug Foscarnet. It is located at 50 Otis Street, Westborough, MA 01581, (508) 366-1100.

asymptomatic   Exhibiting or eliciting no symptoms.

ATEU   *see* AIDS Treatment Evaluation Units

atopic dermatitis   A chronic inflammation of the skin of unknown cause and characterized by severe itching leading to scratching or rubbing, which in turn produces lesions. Individuals affected generally have a hereditary predisposition to irritable skin. *Also called* allergic dermatitis, allergic eczema, and atopic eczema.

atopic diathesis   An allergic condition which makes the body tissues more susceptible to certain diseases.

atopic eczema   *see* atopic dermatitis

ATR   *see* AIDS Treatment Registry

atrophic candidiasis   Infection with a fungus of the genus Candida that causes atrophy. It usually involves the skin or mucous membranes. *See also* atrophy.

atrophy   1) A wasting away; a decrease in the size of a cell, tissue, or organ. 2) To undergo or cause atrophy.

autoimmune mechanism   1) The response that produces antibodies against the body's own tissues. 2) The response that produces the condition in which the body recognizes itself as foreign and forms a humoral and cellular response against the body's own tissues.

autologous transfusion   A transfusion of blood to a patient that has either been donated in advance by the patient or collected at the site of surgery during the procedure. Although current testing procedures have rendered the U.S. blood supply extremely safe, a patient may opt for this procedure because of fear of exposure to the human immunodeficiency virus and other blood-borne infections.

autopsy   An examination of the body after death, including organs and tissues, in order to determine the cause of death or pathological changes. *Also called* necropsy or postmortem examination.

Avlosulfon   *see* dapsone

azathioprine   An immunosuppressive agent, created from a cytotoxic chemical substance and used for the prevention of transplant rejection in organ transplantation. Also under investigation for use in the treatment of autoimmune diseases. The trade name is Imuran.

azidothymidine (AZT)   A synthetic thymidine (one of the basic components of DNA that inhibits the growth and development of the human immunodeficiency virus, which causes the acquired immunodeficiency syndrome. It was the first antiretriviral therapy approved by the Food and Drug Administration. *See also* thymidine.

azotemia   An excess of nitrogenous bodies, especially urea, in the blood. *See also* uremia.

AZT   *see* azidothymidine

AZT failure   Any indication that the condition of a person taking at least 500 mg per day of azidothymidine (AZT) for more than six months is worsening.

AZT ineligibility   Any condition that prohibits a person from taking azidothymidine (AZT), such as low white blood cell count, severe anemia, or administration of incompatible drugs.

AZT intolerance   Any negative, severe side effect resulting from the administration of azidothymidine (AZT) that requires discontinuation of the drug.

B

B cells   *see* B lymphocyte

B lymphocyte   A type of lymphocyte that comes from the bone marrow and is found in the blood, lymph, and connective tissue. When stimulated by an antigen, the B-cell lymphocyte proliferates and differentiates into plasma cells and memory B cells with the cooperation of helper T cells and macrophages. This clone is specific for the antigen for which it was produced.

Bacillus anthracis   An aerobic bacterium belonging to the genus Bacillus. It is the causative agent of anthrax.

bacteremia   The presence of bacteria in the blood.

bacteria   Plural of bacterium.

bacterial infection   The state or condition in which the body or part of it is invaded by bacteria that, under certain conditions, multiply and cause injurious effects.

bacterial pneumonia   Pneumonia caused by bacteria.

bacteriophage   A virus that infects bacteria. They are found throughout nature and have been isolated in excrement, polluted water, and sewage.

bacterium   Any of the unicellular microorganisms of the class Schizomycetes. The organism is usually contained within a cell wall, and multiplication is by cell division (fission). They may be aerobic or anaerobic, motile or nonmotile, and may exist independently, in decaying matter, as parasites, or as pathogens. *See also* gram-negative bacteria and gram-positive bacteria.

Bactrim   *see* trimethoprim/sulfamethoxazole

BAL   *see* bronchoalveolar lavage

Barbados leg   *see* elephantiasis

Baridol   *see* barium sulfate

barium study   1) A test used in examining the gastrointestinal tract. 2) Any test involving the use of barium sulfate as a radiopaque contrast medium (prohibiting the passage of X rays and other forms of radiant energy) for distinguishing anatomical areas in the gastrointestinal tract.

barium sulfate   1) An opaque substance that is swallowed to assist in the examination of the stomach and intestines. 2) An odorless, tasteless, fine, white powder used as a contrast medium in roentgenography (X rays) of the gastrointestinal tract. Trade names are Barosperse, Esophotrast, and Baridol. *Also called* synthetic baryta and blanc fixe.

Barosperse   *see* barium sulfate

Barry, David   Born 1943 in Nashua, N.H. Barry received his M.D. from Yale University School of Medicine in 1969 and is currently Vice President of Research for Burroughs Wellcome. He was instrumental in Wellcome's ability to channel AZT through the Food and Drug Administration for approval and for promoting the drug for treatment of AIDS patients. Burroughs Wellcome Co., 3030 Cornwallis Road, Research Triangle Park, NC 27709, (919) 248-4534.

basal cell carcinoma   A tumor of the skin that rarely metastasizes. It usually manifests as a small, shiny papule. The lesion grows until it appears as a whitish border surrounding a central ulcer.

baseline   A known or initial observation or value used for comparison in measuring the response to experimental intervention or stimulus (e.g., a person's T4-cell count upon entering a clinical trial).

basophil   1) A cell or part of a cell that stains readily with basic dyes. 2) An endocrine found in the anterior lobe of the pituitary gland. It produces the substance that stimulates the adrenal cortex to secrete adrenal cortical hormone. 3) A granular leukocyte character-

ized by the possession of coarse, bluish-black granules of varying size
that stain intensely with basic dyes.

bathhouse   A facility resembling a public bathhouse, but used
primarily for anonymous sexual encounters. Bathhouses came under
heavy fire after it was established that the human immunodeficiency
virus is transmitted through sexual intercourse.

BCG vaccine   A tuberculosis vaccine made from a freeze-dried
preparation of a live strain of Mycobacterium bovis, regularly used
for the vaccination of children only in areas with a high incidence rate
of tuberculosis. In the United States, it is recommended only for
immunizing high-risk persons.

bedsore   *see* decubitus ulcer

benign   1) Not recurrent or progressive. 2) The opposite of
malignant.

beta cell   The cell that secretes insulin and composes the bulk of the
islets of Langerhans.

beta$_2$-microglobulin   A small protein found in human cells that
serves as one subunit of class I major histocompatibility antigens (the
system that has the ability to stimulate an immune response that
causes the rejection of a transplant when a donor and recipient are
mismatched). With HIV infection, beta$_2$ protein is released into the
blood as cells are destroyed by the virus. This may serve as an
indicator that T4 cells are being destroyed and the immune system
weakened.

Bihari, Bernard   Born 1931 in New York City, Bihari received his
M.D. from Harvard Medical School. He was one of the first to detect
AIDS-related infections in drug addicts and one of the original
supporters of the Community Research Initiative. Bihari is currently
a full-time Academic Clinical Associate Professor of Psychiatry at
Downstate Medical Center, Brooklyn, N.Y. Office address: 29 W. 15th
Street, New York, NY 10011, (212) 270-1094.

bilirubin   The orange or yellowish pigment in bile. It is produced by
the degradation of erythrocyte hemoglobin in reticuloendothelial
cells in the bone marrow, the spleen, and elsewhere. It is chemically

altered in the liver and excreted as the water-soluble pigment in the bile. If bilirubin accumulates, it may lead to jaundice.

biomaterial dumping   The sale of a natural or synthetic substance used to replace a bone, tissue, etc., in large quantity at a low price, especially in a foreign market at a price below that of the domestic market.

biopsy   The excision of tissue from a living body for microscopic examination. It is usually performed to establish a diagnosis.

bisexual   An individual exhibiting bisexuality.

bisexuality   1) Sexual attraction to persons of both sexes. 2) Practicing both heterosexual and homosexual behavior.

blackout   1) The sudden loss of consciousness. 2) A condition characterized by a temporary loss of consciousness and failure of vision due to reduced blood circulation to the brain.

blanc fixe   *see* barium sulfate

bleomycin   1) Any of a mixture of antibiotics produced by a strain of Streptomyces verticillus. 2) Any of a group of antitumor antibiotics produced by a strain of Streptomyces verticillus. It is used in conjunction with other chemotherapies for treatment of Hodgkin's disease and non-Hodgkin's lymphomas, squamous cell carcinomas of the head and neck, testicular carcinoma, and uterine cervix carcinoma. Fever, nausea, and vomiting are common side effects. Major side effects include occasionally fatal dose-related pneumonitis, pulmonary fibrosis, and severe skin reactions.

blood products   Anything made naturally or artificially concerning the blood.

blood splash   The accidental scattering of blood so as to wet or soil an individual.

blood supply   The amount of blood stored and available for use.

blood transfusion   The replacement of blood or one of its components.

940724

blow   *see* cocaine

Blue Cross and Blue Shield Association   Founded in 1982, the Association comprises local Blue Cross and Blue Shield Plans for health insurance in the United States, Canada, the United Kingdom, and Jamaica. It works to provide national services through local plans, promote improvement of public health, and secure public acceptance of health insurance services. The Association produces various publications, and has an on-site library. Blue Cross and Blue Shield Association, 676 N. St. Clair Street, Chicago, IL 60611, (312) 440-6000.

BLV   *see* bovine leukemia virus

bodily fluid   Any of the liquids contained in or produced by the human body (e.g., blood, perspiration, saliva, semen, tears, vaginal secretions). *Also called* body fluid.

body fluid   *see* bodily fluid

boil   *see* furuncle

Bolognesi, Dani Paul   Born 1941 in Forgaria, Italy, Bolognesi received his Ph.D. in virology from Duke University in 1967. A prominent virologist, he has been a leader in studying the structure of the human immunodeficiency virus and assisted with the testing of AZT. Bolognesi is Professor of Surgery and Associate Professor of Microbiology/Immunology, Duke University Medical Center. Department of Surgery, Duke University Medical Center, P.O. Box 2926, Durham, NC 27710.

bone marrow suppression   Any chemical or process that suppresses the production of cells or the maturation of cells within the bone marrow.

booting   The procedure practiced by intravenous drug users in which blood is withdrawn into the drug-filled syringe prior to injecting the entire contents. The process is supposed to enhance the drug-induced high. Booting increases the risk for transmission of the human immunodeficiency virus by providing increased contact between the blood and the syringe.

bootleg   To produce, carry, or sell illegally.

bovine leukemia virus   A virus found in cattle that is similar in structure to the human T-cell leukemia virus.

brachioproctic eroticism   Penetration of the rectum with the hand and forearm to induce sexual stimulation. *Also called* fisting or fist-fucking.

brain imaging   The use of X ray or nuclear techniques that produce an image representative of the brain.

brain scan   The process used to detect aberrations in the function or structure of the brain by injecting radioactive isotopes into the circulatory system.

breast-feeding   The nursing of an infant at a mother's breast.

Bristol-Myers Squibb Company   A pharmaceutical company that holds the license for dideoxyinosine (ddI), and other health care products. The main office is located at 345 Park Avenue, New York, NY 10154, (212) 546-4000.

broad-spectrum   Effective against a variety of microorganisms.

Broder, Samuel   Born 1945, Broder received his M.D. from the University of Michigan Medical School in 1970. He was one of the investigators responsible for AZT. Broder is the Director of the National Cancer Institute Clinical Center. National Cancer Institute, 9000 Rockville Pike, Bethesda, MD 20892, (301) 496-5615.

bronchi   Plural of bronchus.

bronchoalveolar lavage (BAL)   The washing out of the bronchus and alveoli to remove irritants, or to diagnose inflammation or infection.

bronchoscopy   A procedure to examine the bronchi in which an instrument, a bronchoscope, is inserted orally for the purpose of taking specimens for culture and biopsy. It is used to diagnose pulmonary disorders such as Pneumocystis carinii pneumonia.

bronchus   1) Any of the larger air passages of the lungs. 2) One of the large branches of the trachea.

brush biopsy   A biopsy in which tiny brushes are used to remove cells or tissue.

budding   A method of asexual reproduction in which a budlike appendage grows from the side or end of the parent and develops into a new organism (the larger part is considered the parent and the smaller one the bud). The bud may remain attached, or separate and live independently of the parent. This form of reproduction is common in lower animals and plants, including many of the fungi that invade the human body.

Burkitt's lymphoma   1) A form of cancer characterized most often by tumors in the jaw or abdominal area. 2) A form of highly undifferentiated lymphoblastic lymphoma manifested most often in the jaw or as an abdominal mass. It involves sites other than the lymph nodes and reticuloendothelial system. This form of lymphoma is rare in the United States and is found most commonly in Central Africa. The Epstein-Barr virus has been implicated as the causative agent.

Burroughs Wellcome Company   A pharmaceutical company that includes AZT among its products. It is located at 3030 Cornwallis Road, Research Triangle Park, NC 27709, (919) 248-3000.

Busse-Buschke disease   *see* cryptococcosis

butyl nitrite inhalant   A liquid compound that dilates blood vessels and reduces blood pressure when inhaled. It is used recreationally to produce a brief high. Unlike amyl nitrite, butyl nitrite does not require a prescription. *Also called* rush and poppers.

buyers' club   *see* buyers' group

buyers' group   A group that imports from other countries drugs not yet approved for use in the United States by the Food and Drug Administration. *Also called* buyers' club.

C

CAIDS *see* Community Acquired Immune Deficiency Syndrome

CAIN *see* Computerized AIDS Information Network

Calcium Folinate *see* folinic acid

Callen, Michael One of the founders of the People With AIDS Coalition and two now-defunct New York groups, Gay Men With AIDS and PWA-New York. Callen is an author, singer, and advocate for community-based AIDS research and is a long-time survivor with AIDS.

Campbell, Bobbi One of the first persons in San Francisco to be diagnosed with Kaposi's sarcoma and to make his diagnosis public. In 1981, Campbell dubbed himself the "KS Poster Boy." He was instrumental in starting the National Association of People With AIDS.

Campylobacter 1) A genus of bacteria that is a cause of diarrhea in AIDS patients. 2) A genus of bacteria made up of gram-negative, non-spore-forming, spiral shaped, motile rods with polar flagella. These bacteria are found in both humans and animals in the intestinal tract, oral cavity, and reproductive systems. Certain species are pathogenic and may cause enteritis or systemic disease in humans, and abortion in some animals.

CAN *see* Cure AIDS Now

cancer 1) A harmful new growth anywhere in the body. 2) A malignant tumor. Cancer cells possess the properties of invasion and metastasis and comprise a broad group of neoplasms. These are divided into two groups: carcinoma (those originating in epithelial tissues) and sarcoma (those developing from connective tissues and structures having their origin in mesodermal tissues).

Candida   1) A fungus that is a common cause of opportunistic infections in people with AIDS. 2) A genus of yeastlike fungi that is characterized by the production of yeast cells. Reproduction is performed by budding. It is commonly part of the flora of the mouth, skin, intestinal tract, and vagina. Candida may cause a variety of infections such as candidiasis or vaginitis.

candidal endocarditis   Infection of the internal lining or structures of the heart with fungi of the genus Candida.

candidemia   The presence of fungi of the genus Candida in the blood. This condition usually results from systemic candidiasis or candidal endocarditis.

candidiasis   1) A fungal infection that occurs in several places in the body, including the mouth or throat (thrush), vagina, and on the skin; a common opportunistic infection in people with AIDS. 2) Infection with a fungus of the genus Candida. It usually infects the moist cutaneous areas of the body (skin or mucous membranes) and is chiefly caused by Candida albicans. *Also called* candidosis, oidomycosis, and moniliasis.

candidosis   *see* candidiasis

carcinoma   1) Any of several kinds of cancerous growths made up of epithelial cells. 2) A new growth or malignant tumor made up of epithelial cells. These neoplasms tend to infiltrate the surrounding tissue and give rise to metastases. It may affect almost any part of the body or its organs.

cardiovascular syphilis   1) Syphilis involving the heart and great blood vessels. 2) A form of tertiary syphilis involving the heart and great blood vessels, especially the aorta. Aortic aneurysms and aortic insufficiency often result, thereby causing damage to the intima and media of the great blood vessels. Congestive heart failure may result.

caregiver   An individual charged with or assuming the responsibility of watching over or attending to a physically or mentally ill person.

case-doubling time   The amount of time necessary for the occurrence of a disease to double in number.

case history   The collection of data concerning an individual regarding his/her medical, family, psychiatric, and social history. This information is gathered to provide a better understanding of the patient and is useful in analyzing and diagnosing the present illness.

case management   The handling of an individual incidence of disease, injury, or other medical abnormality, with the result being care and/or treatment that is satisfactory under the circumstances.

casual social contact   1) The act or state of occasionally or superficially meeting or touching someone. 2) Interpersonal contact that is not intimate.

CAT scan   *see* computerized axial tomographic scan

cat-scratch disease   An infectious disease that is transmitted by the bite or scratch of a cat. It is caused by Pasteurella multocida. The disease is characterized by the formation of an abscess at the site of infection followed by enlargement of nearby lymph nodes.

cathartic   1) Causing purgation of the bowels. 2) A purgative agent that causes evacuation of the bowels.

cavitary lesion   1) A circumscribed area of tissue altered by disease and characterized by the formation of a cavity. 2) Any lesion characterized by cavitation (internal or central necrosis), such as cavitary tuberculous.

cavitation   1) Formation of a cavity. 2) A cavity.

CCA   *see* Citizens Commission on AIDS

CCBC   *see* Council of Community Blood Centers

CDC   *see* Centers for Disease Control and Prevention

cefotaxime   1) A broad-spectrum antibiotic. 2) A third generation cephalosporin that is a semisynthetic derivative of cephamycin and is effective against gram-negative organisms that have the ability to resist certain types of antibiotics such as penicillin.

CEH   *see* Center for Environmental Health

cellular immunity   1) Immunity mediated by T lymphocytes. 2) T-cell-mediated immune functions that need cell interactions (i.e., the destruction of infected cells).

Center for Environmental Health (CEH)   One of the nine major components of the Centers for Disease Control and Prevention. It is concerned with the control of environmentally related diseases and chronic diseases. Center for Environmental Health, Centers for Disease Control and Prevention, Department of Health and Human Services, Public Health Service, 1600 Clifton Road, N.E., Atlanta, GA 30333, (404) 452-4111.

Center for Infectious Diseases (CID)   One of the nine major components of the Centers for Disease Control and Prevention. It is concerned with the identification, diagnosis, prevention, and control of infectious diseases. Center for Infectious Diseases, Centers for Disease Control and Prevention, Department of Health and Human Services, Public Health Service, 1600 Clifton Road, N.E., Atlanta, GA 30333, (404) 329-3401.

Centers for Disease Control and Prevention (CDC)   The Federal agency operating under the U.S. Department of Health and Human Services, Public Health Service, that is responsible for protecting the public health of the nation by instituting measures for the prevention and control of diseases, epidemics, and public health emergencies. Founded in 1946. Centers for Disease Control and Prevention, Department of Health and Human Services, Public Health Service, 1600 Clifton Road, N.E., Atlanta, GA 30333, (404) 639-3286.

central nervous system (CNS)   The part of the body consisting of the brain and spinal cord, along with their nerves and ends of nerve fibers, that controls voluntary and involuntary muscles. It includes control of consciousness and mental functioning, sensory organs, and skeletal muscles.

central spinal fluid (CSF)   *see* cerebrospinal fluid

cerebrospinal fluid   The watery liquid that serves as a buffer to protect the brain and spinal cord from physical impact. *Also called* central spinal fluid or CSF.

cerebrovascular accident (CVA)   A general term applied to conditions concerning the blood vessels of the brain that accompany either ischemic (caused by a lack of blood supply) or hemorrhagic (caused by the escape of large quantities of blood) lesions. *Also called* apoplexy or stroke.

cervical cancer   Cancer of the cervix uteri.

cervical secretion   Any material produced by the cervix uteri from the blood.

cervix   1) The neck, or part of an organ resembling a neck such as a collum. 2) The lower part of the uterus, extending to the vagina.

cervix uteri   The neck of the uterus.

chancre   The primary ulcer of syphilis, usually hard and painless, which appears at the point at which the infection enters the body. The lesion begins as an erosion or papule which is red or raw in color. It exudes fluid and continues to indurate. The sore heals without scarring. Syphilis is highly contagious during the chancre stage.

charbon   *see* anthrax

chemotaxis   The movement of cells in response to a chemical signal or stimulus (e.g., the movement of macrophages to the site of an inflammatory reaction).

chemotherapy   The treatment of disease by chemical reagents that have a toxic effect upon the disease-causing microorganism.

chest radiograph   An X ray film of the chest cavity, taken for the purpose of making a definitive observation or measurement.

child   Any human between infancy and puberty.

Chlamydia   1) A genus of bacteria that cause a variety of diseases in humans and other animals. 2) A genus of obligate, intracellular parasites that cause a variety of diseases in humans and animals. One species (Chlamydia trachomatis) has been recognized as a major sexually transmitted and perinatal infection, with genital infections caused by Chlamydia trachomatis being the most common sexually transmitted disease in the United States.

chlamydia   Any member of the genus Chlamydia.

chloramphenicol   A synthetic, broad-spectrum antibiotic that was originally isolated from Streptomyces venezuelae. It appears as elongated, needle-shaped crystals, and is whitish, grayish, or yellowish in color. It is especially useful in the treatment of typhus and other rickettsial infections, shigellosis, typhoid fever (for which it is the primary antibiotic for treatment), and salmonellosis (an opportunistic infectious complication of AIDS). In the treatment of bacterial infections, chloramphenicol may be administered orally or applied topically. It is administered orally in the treatment of rickettsial infections. Trade names are Chloromycetin and Chloroptic.

Chloromycetin   *see* chloramphenicol

Chloroptic   *see* chloramphenicol

cholera   An acute infection of the small intestine characterized by vomiting and painless, watery diarrhea, which results in the depletion of fluids and electrolytes, dehydration, muscular cramps, faint high-pitched voice, and collapse. Cholera is spread by feces-contaminated food and water. It is common in India and Southeast Africa, spreading periodically to other parts of the world.

chorioid   *see* choroid

chorioidea   *see* choroid

chorioretinitis   Inflammation of the choroid and retina. *Also called* retinochoroiditis.

choroid   The thin, dark brown, vascular coat of the eye that extends from the ora serrata to the optic nerve. It consists of blood vessels and connective tissue that furnish the blood supply to the retina. *Also called* chorioid, chorioidea, and choroidea.

choroidea   *see* choroid

chronic   1) Persisting over a long period of time. 2) Designating a disease exhibiting a slow progression. 3) The opposite of acute.

chronic ambulatory peritoneal dialysis   A treatment for kidney failure. Dialysis prolonged over a period of time in which warm, sterile, chemical solutions are perfused through the lining of the peritoneal cavity in order to remove toxic substances from the body. The patient is not confined to bed, and the procedure is usually repeated several times daily for as long as kidney function remains severely impaired.

chronic hyperplastic candidiasis   Infection of the skin or mucous membrane with a species of Candida that causes a slow, excessive proliferation of normal cells in the normal tissue arrangement of the infected organ.

chronic infection   The invasion by, and multiplication of, a pathogenic agent in the body that persists over a prolonged period of time producing injurious effects.

chronic vaginal yeast infection   Infection of the vagina by any of several unicellular fungi of the genus saccharomyces that persists over a prolonged period of time.

CID   *see* Center for Infectious Diseases

Citizens Commission on AIDS (CCA)   Founded in 1987, this organization consisted of executives, leaders, and officials from the public and private sector concerned with the impact of HIV and AIDS on society. It sought to study and develop policies regarding the epidemic and to address the various ethical, moral, and legal aspects associated with the disease. The Project ended in 1991 with the production of a final report.

citrovorum factor   *see* folinic acid

cleocin   *see* clindamycin

clindamycin   An antibiotic that is effective against gram-positive bacteria and some anaerobic infections. It has been used effectively to treat chorioretinitis. It has also been suggested that clindamycin used in conjunction with other drugs such as pyrimethamine may be successful treatment for infection with Toxoplasma gondii in some patients. The trade name is Cleocin.

clinical trial   A carefully designed and administered investigation of the effects of a new drug on human subjects. The purpose of a trial is to establish the clinical efficacy, safety, and pharmacologic effects of the substance. This is the process through which new drugs must pass in order to be approved by the United States Food and Drug Administration. *See also* parallel track.

clofazimine   An antibacterial that is used in the treatment of leprosy and tuberculosis.

clone   1) A genetically identical offspring of a cell, organism, or plant propagated through asexual reproduction from a single parent. 2) To form a clone.

cloning   The process of forming a clone.

clotrimazole   A broad-spectrum, antifungal drug used in the treatment of candidiasis and tinea. It is applied topically to the affected area of the skin or intravaginally in the treatment of vulvovaginal candidiasis. Trade names include Gyne-Lotrimin, Lotrimin, and Mycelex G.

CMV retinitis   *see* cytomegalovirus retinitis

Cnidosporidia   *see* Microsporida

CNS   *see* central nervous system

cocaine   A crystalline alkaloid obtained from the leaves of the shrub Erythroxylon coca and other Erythroxylon species. Cocaine may be used as a narcotic anesthetic when applied topically to mucous membranes. When administered for non-medical use, it is classed as a drug of abuse. It may also be produced synthetically. *Also called* blow, coke, and toot.

Coccidia   A large order of parasitic protozoa found in both vertebrates and invertebrates. They generally infect epithelial cells of the intestine and associated glands and are the causative agent of coccidiosis.

Coccidioides   1) A genus of fungi found in the soils of the southwestern United States that frequently infect persons with AIDS from this area. 2) A genus of imperfect, pathogenic fungi with a single species, Coccidioides immitis. Coccidioides immitis is the causative agent of coccidioidomycosis. *See also* coccidioidomycosis.

Coccidioides immitis   *see* Coccidioides

coccidioidomycosis   A fungal disease caused by infection with Coccidioides immitis. It exists in two forms: primary (an acute, self-limiting disease involving the respiratory system) and secondary or progressive (a chronic, severe, virulent, tumor-containing disease that may involve almost any part of the body).

coccidiosis   A disease-producing condition caused by infection with coccidia generally affecting the intestines. In humans, symptoms include watery, mucous stools; anorexia; and nausea.

code-blue status   Directions to employ active and aggressive cardiopulmonary resuscitation in the event of the apparent cessation of life.

cofactor   An element or principle that acts in conjunction with another. Generally, the cofactor must be present for the other to function.

cognition   The mental process by which one becomes aware of thought and perception, including reasoning, judgment, and memory.

coke   *see* cocaine

colitis   Inflammation of the colon.

coloproctitis   *see* proctocolitis

Community Acquired Immune Deficiency Syndrome (CAIDS)   One of a group of names initially used to denote the acquired immunodeficiency syndrome. *See also* gay-related immune deficiency, acquired community immune deficiency syndrome, and acquired immunodeficiency syndrome.

Community Research Initiative (CRI)   The first community organization to do actual drug research on possible treatments for AIDS and the various diseases and opportunistic infections that accompany it. The program is now part of the People With AIDS Coalition. Community Research Initiative, People With AIDS Coalition, 31 W. 26th Street, New York, NY 10011, (212) 532-0290.

Compassionate Use   A program developed by the Food and Drug Administration to supply experimental drugs to the seriously ill who have no other alternatives. Compassionate use allows a drug to be dispensed in lieu of following the standard protocol for FDA approval (clinical trials).

competence   The condition or quality to manage one's affairs; the ability to fulfill one's needs.

complement fixation test   A procedure used to detect antigens or antibodies. Complement fixation involves the action of a complement upon reaction with immune complexes containing complement-fixing antibodies. The complement is rendered inactive during the uniting of antibody, antigen, and complement (fixation of complement). This is the basis for determining the presence of antigens or antibodies.

Compound Q   *see* GLQ-223

computed tomographic scan   *see* computerized axial tomographic scan

Computerized AIDS Information Network (CAIN)   An electronic information system designed for health care professionals and individuals concerned with AIDS education. In addition to bibliographic and factual information (clinical data, service providers, organization assistance, information resources), the system includes an electronic bulletin board, computer conferencing, and electronic mail. It is produced by the Gay and Lesbian Community Service Center, CAIN, 1213 N. Highland Avenue, Hollywood, CA 90038, (213) 464-7400, ext. 277.

computerized axial tomographic (CAT) scan   1) A noninvasive procedure for diagnosing disorders of the body, especially in the soft tissues, using special X-ray techniques. 2) A noninvasive procedure employing special techniques of roentgenography in which transverse planes of tissue are swept by an X-ray beam and the variance in absorption is recorded on a magnetic disk, processed on a minicomputer, and used to produce a precise reconstruction of that area. This technique is more sensitive than traditional radiographic procedures and has been very successful in diagnostic studies of the brain. *Also called* CAT scan and computed tomographic scan.

Conant, Marcus   Born 1936 in Jacksonville, Fla., Conant received his M.D. from Duke University in 1961. He began diagnosing Kaposi's sarcoma in persons with AIDS early in the epidemic. Conant has a private practice and is a Clinical Professor of Dermatology at the University of California, San Francisco. Office address: 350 Parnassus Street, San Francisco, CA 94117, (415) 661-2613.

condom   A thin, flexible sheath or cover for the penis worn during sexual intercourse to prevent semen from entering the mouth, anus, or vagina and to prevent venereal disease. Only condoms made of latex are considered effective in helping to prevent transmission of the human immunodeficiency virus.

condyloma acuminatum   1) A wart occurring on the area around the anus or external genitals. 2) A papilloma caused by a virus and occurring on the mucous membrane or skin of the external genitals or perianal region. It is infectious and autoinoculable. Although the lesions are usually small in number, they may cluster to form a cauliflower-like mass. *Also called* venereal wart.

confidentiality   The privacy afforded information entrusted to health care and other professionals concerning a patient (e.g., test results).

congenital   Existing at birth; present at birth.

conservatorship   The responsibility or rank of custodian, guardian, or protector.

contact tracing   The practice of following the track of individuals who have been recently exposed to a contagious disease; implies informing those individuals who may have been exposed.

contraceptive   An agent, device, method, or process that works to prevent conception (pregnancy). Common classes include chemical (spermicides, birth control pills), natural (abstinence, rhythm), physical or barrier (condoms, IUDs, sponges, caps, diaphragms), and permanent (tubal ligation, vasectomy).

control group   A group of persons representing a standard against which observations or conclusions may be compared for the purpose of verifying the results of an experiment. The control group functions as a means of isolating the variable being studied by allowing other factors to be matched with those of the experimental group. In an experiment testing the efficacy of a drug, the control group would be the persons not receiving the drug being studied.

Coomb's-positive anemia   Any type of anemia detected by a Coomb's test.

Coomb's test   A procedure used to detect antiglobulins in the red cell. It is used in diagnosing various hemolytic anemias.

correctional institution   Any facility charged with carrying out punishment for the purpose of altering behavior (e.g., juvenile detention center or prison).

corticosteroid   Any of the hormonal steroids obtained from the adrenal cortex. Divided as to their biological activity into 3 main groups: glucocorticoids (those affecting carbohydrate, fat, and protein metabolism), mineralocorticoids (those influencing the regulation of electrolyte and water balance), and androgen (those affecting the development of male characteristics). Corticosteroids do not initiate activity but allow for many biochemical reactions to proceed at optimal rates.

cortisone   A hormone found in the cortex of the adrenal gland and also produced synthetically. It is useful in the treatment of various allergic, inflammatory, and neoplastic diseases.

Corynebacterium infantisepticum   *see* Listeria monocytogenes

Corynebacterium parvulum   *see* Listeria monocytogenes

Cotinazin   *see* isoniazid

cotton-wool spots   Fluffy white lesions with obvious boundaries that appear on the eye. These are generally not associated with hemorrhages and should be differentiated from cytomegalovirus retinitis, since they are generally asymptomatic, they may subside voluntarily, and prognosis is usually excellent.

Council of Community Blood Centers (CCBC)   Founded in 1962, this organization comprises nonprofit, independent blood centers licensed by the federal government and serving specific geographic areas. It serves to ensure the maintenance and provision of an optimal supply of blood and blood products. The CCBC conducts research, compiles statistics, and serves as a liaison to various organizations interested in the storage of blood. Council of Community Blood Centers, 725 15th Street, N.W., Suite 700, Washington, DC 20005, (202) 393-5725.

counseling   The provision of advice or guidance to a patient by health care and other professionals. Counseling is often recommended to assist a patient in coping with stress or working through various types of problems.

cranial nerve palsy   The temporary or permanent loss of sensation, or ability to control movement, in the twelve pairs of nerves that originate in the brain.

craniofacial feature   The appearance, form, or shape of the face and the skeleton of the head.

Creutzfeldt-Jakob disease   A rare, transmissible, usually fatal disease that causes degeneration of the brain. It is accompanied by progressive dementia and sometimes wasting of the muscles, tremor, and spastic speech impairment. The way the disease is acquired naturally is unknown; however, human-to-human transmission has occurred by parenteral administration of growth hormone prepared from cadaveric human pituitary glands, cadaveric dura mater graft, implantation of contaminated electroencephalographic electrodes, and corneal transplantation.

CRI   *see* Community Research Initiative

crisis intervention   The process of alleviating or terminating an unstable emotional or mental period in a person's life through problem resolution. Many telephone hotlines (e.g., suicide prevention or AIDS hotlines) function as crisis intervention services.

cryptococcosis   1) A serious opportunistic fungal infection by Cryptococcus neoformans that may involve several places in the body. 2) A systemic infection by Cryptococcus neoformans that may involve the skin, lungs, or any organ of the body, but has a predilection for the brain and meninges. The cutaneous form is characterized by abscesses or lesions. In the generalized form, the central nervous system is the primary target for attack. This is marked by dizziness, headache, stiffness of the neck muscles, and vertigo. If untreated, coma and respiratory failure result. *Also called* Busse-Buschke disease and torulosis.

Cryptococcus   A genus of asexual, pathogenic, yeastlike fungi. Cryptococcus neoformans is the causative agent of cryptococcosis.

cryptosporidiosis   An enteric (gastrointestinal) disease caused by infection with protozoa of the genus cryptosporidium and characterized by diarrhea. This disease is not uncommon in hoofed animals. Human occurrence appears in both the immunocompetent and immunocompromised. Among the immunocompetent, infection is largely among those working with infected animals. For these individuals, diarrhea is accompanied by abdominal cramps and lasts up to a month. The malady is self-limiting, and there is no therapy. The disease is much more serious in the immunocompromised patient and often results in death. Diarrhea is prolonged and debilitating; it is accompanied by abdominal cramps, fever, and weight loss.

Cryptosporidium   A genus of parasitic, coccidian protozoa. They inhabit the intestinal tracts of various birds, mammals, and reptiles. In humans, infection may cause diarrhea. This is especially true for the immunocompromised patient. *See also* cryptosporidiosis.

CSF   *see* cerebrospinal fluid

culture   1) The propagation of microorganisms or of living tissue cells in special media that are conducive to their growth. 2) The ideas, beliefs, and customs of a group of people that are transferred or communicated to subsequent generations.

Cumulated Index Medicus   An annual index, updated monthly, to biomedical literature. It is produced by the National Library of Medicine, and citations are compiled from the vast collection of journals collected by the library. *Also called* Index Medicus. MEDLINE is the electronic counterpart. National Library of Medicine, 8600 Rockville Pike, Bethesda, MD 20894.

cunnilingus   Sexual activity in which the female genitalia are stimulated with the tongue and mouth.

Cure AIDS Now (CAN)   Founded in 1985, this organization seeks to educate the public about the reality and gravity of the AIDS pandemic. It also functions as a support network for persons with

AIDS and for those interested in assisting with the fight to stop the spread of HIV. CAN also coordinates resources donated by private and corporate sources to create and execute AIDS assistance programs. Cure AIDS Now, 2240 S. Dixie Highway, Coconut Grove, FL 33133, (305) 856-TEST.

Curran, James W.   Born 1944 in Monroe, Mich., Curran received his M.D. from the University of Michigan in 1970, and his M.P.H. from the School of Public Health, Harvard University, in 1974. He is the Director of the WHO Reference Center for AIDS and Retroviruses. Center for Infectious Diseases, AIDS Program, Centers for Disease Control and Prevention, 1600 Clifton Road, N.E., Building 6-288, Atlanta, GA 30333.

cutaneous abnormalities   A malformation or deformity of the skin.

cutaneous Kaposi's sarcoma   Kaposi's sarcoma of the skin.

CVA   *see* cerebrovascular accident

cycloserine   A broad-spectrum antibiotic administered orally and shown to be effective in the treatment of tuberculosis. It is also effective against various gram-positive and gram-negative bacteria, including some that infect the pulmonary system and urinary tract. The trade name is Seromycin.

cyclosporine A   An immunosuppressive and antifungal drug used to prevent rejection in organ transplant recipients. The trade name is Sandimmune.

cytokine   1) A substance that is released by a cell population when it is stimulated by a specific antigen. 2) A nonantibody protein that is released when a specific antigen interacts with a cell population. Cytokines serve as the substance situated between cells that enables the generation and propagation amplification of a response. (Example: T-lymphocytes emit cytokines, allowing for an immune response.)

cytomegalic inclusion disease   Any of a group of diseases caused by infection with the cytomegalovirus and marked by the presence of bodies in the cytoplasm of infected cells. Infection can occur congenitally; postnatally; via respiratory droplets; from infected transplanted tissue or transfused blood; or through sexual intercourse. Included in this group is an infectious mononucleosis-like syndrome that occurs in recipients of multiple blood transfusions and previously well individuals and a disseminated infection in immunosuppressed or immunocompromised patients that is fatal.

cytomegalovirus (CMV)   One of a group of highly species-specific herpesviruses that infect humans, monkeys, and rodents. In humans, cytomegalovirus is found in the salivary glands. It may cause a variety of clinical syndromes that are collectively known as cytomegalic inclusion disease. *Also called* salivary gland virus.

cytomegalovirus retinitis (CMV retinitis)   Inflammation of the retina, which may result in blindness, due to infection with the cytomegalovirus.

cytotoxicity   The degree to which an agent possesses a specific property that is destructive to certain cells.

D

dapsone 1) A broad-spectrum antibacterial. 2) An antibacterial sulfone administered orally and used in the treatment of leprosy that inhibits or retards bacterial growth in a variety of gram-negative and gram-positive organisms. Also used in the treatment of dermatitis herpetiformis and in the prophylaxis of falciparum malaria and Pneumocystis carinii pneumonia. *Also called* diaminodiphenylsulfone or DDS. The trade name is Avlosulfon.

dapsone/trimethoprim Combination drug therapy using dapsone and trimethoprim. A common outpatient regimen for the treatment of Pneumocystis carinii pneumonia.

Daraprim *see* pyrimethamine

ddC *see* dideoxycytidine

ddI *see* dideoxyinosine

DDS *see* dapsone

death with dignity The concept of allowing a patient to die, rather than artificially prolonging his or her life, that arose out of the ability of modern medical and technological advances to maintain vital functions in persons who might otherwise die.

decubitus ulcer 1) A bedsore. 2) An ulceration of the skin due to prolonged pressure over the affected area in a patient allowed to lie still in the same position in bed too long. The tissue dies due to a lack of blood supply. Areas with prominent bones are at greatest risk. If not treated properly, the ulcer can progress to the deeper layers of the skin and may eventually affect the underlying muscle and bone.

definitive diagnosis   1) A diagnosis established with certainty, without question. 2) The opposite of presumptive diagnosis.

Delaney, Martin   An AIDS activist and founder of Project Inform. Diagnosed with chronic hepatitis in 1980, he enrolled in an experimental drug treatment program at Stanford University. The drugs stopped the liver deterioration but left him with a severe neuropathy. The experimental program was stopped in 1982, with several participants dying after cessation of treatment. Delaney went on to build a successful consulting business. In 1985 he used his skills to set up Project Inform, a service for the gathering and disseminating of data concerning treatments for AIDS. Delaney is currently the Director of Project Inform. Project Inform, 347 Dolores Street, Suite 301, San Francisco, CA 94110, (800) 822-7422.

delirium   A state of mental confusion and disorder characterized by the inability to focus attention, disorientation, incoherent speech, sensory misperceptions, disturbance in motor skills, and memory impairment. Forms of delirium vary depending on the cause (infection, fever, drug overdose or side effect, shock, trauma, or metabolic disturbances).

deltacortisone   *see* prednisone

Deltasone   *see* prednisone

demography   The statistical and quantitative science dealing with the age, density, distribution, growth, size, and vital statistics of human populations.

demyelinate   To remove or destroy the myelin sheath surrounding a nerve or nerves, interrupting the transmission of nerve impulses.

dendrite   One of the threadlike extensions of the cytoplasm of a neuron that comprise most of its receptive surface and conduct impulses to another nerve cell body.

denial   1) A defense mechanism in which the existence of anxiety-producing realities are kept out of conscious awareness. 2) The refusal to admit the existence of something.

dental dam   A barrier, usually of latex or plastic, used primarily in oral-vaginal sex to prevent vaginal secretions from entering the mouth.

deoxynojirimycin   A plant alkaloid that, in the laboratory, inhibits cell-to-cell spread and formation of nucleated protoplasmic mass induced by the human immunodeficiency virus.

deoxyribonucleic acid (DNA)   A nucleic acid that makes up the genetic material of cellular organisms and DNA viruses. It is a complex protein, high in molecular weight, consisting of deoxyribose, phosphoric acid, and four bases [two purines (adenine and guanine) and two pyrimides (thymine and cytosine)]. It is bound by hydrogen bonds between the bases into double helical chains, forming the basic material in the chromosomes of the cell nucleus.

Department of Health and Human Services   The U.S. government's cabinet-level department most involved with the nation's human concerns. Department of Health and Human Services, 200 Independence Avenue, S.W., Washington, DC 20201, (202) 619-0257.

depression   1) A hollow or concave region. 2) A decrease or lowering of a functional activity or vital function. 3) A mental state denoted by an altered mood and characterized by feelings of despair, discouragement, guilt, hopelessness, helplessness, the inability to cope, low self-esteem, and sadness. Depression often results in withdrawal from those activities usually found to be pleasurable. It may also cause changes in eating patterns, energy, and sleep disturbances and ranges from a general feeling of the blues to major clinical depression.

dermatitis   Inflammation of the skin.

dermatitis medicamentosa   *see* drug eruption

Design Industries Foundation For AIDS (DIFFA)   A national grantmaking foundation begun in 1984 that encompasses fashion, textile, visual display, tabletop, exhibit, floral, product, hospitality, and craft design as well as the design publishing community. Through DIFFA, grants are awarded to organizations that provide direct-care services to people with HIV and AIDS, AIDS education and awareness, and public policy and advocacy. DIFFA, 150 W. 26th Street, Suite 602, New York, NY 10001, (212) 727-3100.

Designated AIDS Center Program   A program created and implemented by the New York State Department of Health (funded by Medicaid to cover New York) to assist with the high cost of AIDS care and treatment. It seeks to help by addressing the ways in which health care services are organized. *See also* AIDS Health Service Program, AIDS Service Demonstration Program, and AIDS-specific Medicaid Home and Community-Based Waiver.

desmopressin   A vasopressin analogue with antidiuretic (water retention) properties used in the treatment of diabetes insipidus. Also used to increase Factor VIII (the factor contributing to the intrinsic value of blood coagulation) for hemophiliacs or patients with von Willebrand's disease before surgery.

DeVita, Vincent T., Jr.   Born 1935 in Bronx, N.Y., DeVita received his M.D. from George Washington University School of Medicine in 1961. He was the director of the National Cancer Institute when the acquired immunodeficiency syndrome was first identified. Currently a Professor of Medicine at the Medical College, Cornell University, DeVita is an attending physician, Department of Medicine, Memorial Sloan-Kettering Cancer Center, 1275 York Avenue, New York, NY 10021, (212) 639-5842.

dextran sulfate   1) A potential treatment for HIV infection that proved to be ineffective. 2) A sulfated polysaccharide that showed promise as an antiviral treatment for HIV infection in vitro, but in a Phase I/II trial in San Francisco demonstrated no antiviral or clinical immunological efficacy.

DHPG   *see* ganciclovir

diabetes insipidus   A metabolic disorder caused by damage to the neurohypophyseal system (the main portion of the posterior lobe of the pituitary gland). This results in deficient amounts of antidiuretic hormone (vasopressin) produced or released. As a result, the individual experiences uncontrollable excessive thirst and urination. It may be acquired, inherited, or of unknown origin.

diacetylmorphine   A narcotic morphine derivative that appears as a white, crystalline powder. Because of its highly addictive nature, importation, use, and sale are illegal in the United States. *Also called* heroin.

diagnosis   The use of scientific methods to determine the cause and nature of a person's disease or illness.

dialysis   The process of separating out materials in solution due to the difference in their rates of diffusion through a semipermeable membrane. *See also* hemodialysis and peritoneal dialysis.

diaminodiphenylsulfone   *see* dapsone

diarrhea   A disturbance in bowel movements characterized by abnormal frequency and liquidity. Diarrhea is often related to a disturbance in the gastrointestinal system.

diarrhea-wasting syndrome   A term sometimes used to refer to diarrhea as commonly associated with HIV infection. The syndrome (diarrhea persisting for at least 1 month accompanied by unexplained weight loss of 10% of the premorbid weight) in conjunction with infection with the human immunodeficiency virus comprises an AIDS-defining illness.

didanosine   *see* dideoxyinosine

dideoxycytidine (ddC)   A nucleoside analogue similar to zidovudine but exhibiting less toxicity. Trade name is HIVID.

dideoxyinosine (ddI)   A nucleoside analogue similar to zidovudine. Trade name is Videx.

DIFFA   *see* Design Industries Foundation For AIDS

differential diagnosis   The diagnostic approach that compares the symptoms of two or more similar diseases in order to determine which one the patient is suffering from.

dihydroxypropoxymethyl (DHPG)   *see* gancyclovir

diiodohydroxyquin   *see* iodoquinol

Dinacrin   *see* isoniazid

Diodoquin   *see* iodoquinol

dipstick test   A method to determine the presence of protein, glucose, or other substances in the urine using a chemically impregnated strip of paper.

discrimination   The process of differentiation, distinguishing, or exclusion based on some characteristic or trait (e.g., racial, religious, sexual).

disinfection   The act of freeing from pathogenic organisms, or rendering them inactive, by physical or chemical means. Generally used in reference to inanimate objects.

disseminated tuberculosis   Mycobacterium tuberculosis that has spread from the primary focus of infection through the blood or lymphatic system.

distal   Remote; away from the point of origin.

distal symmetric polyneuropathy (DSPN)   A disease of the nerves that manifests as subacute onset of numbness or tingling in the fingers or toes. Early clinical signs are bilaterally depressed ankle reflex and impaired sensation in the toes. Approximately 35 percent of hospitalized AIDS patients are affected by DSPN.

DNA   *see* deoxyribonucleic acid

DNA polymerase alpha   An enzyme essential to the life of a cell for its synthetic and repair functions.

DNA polymerase beta   An enzyme with repair functions in the life of a cell.

DNA polymerase gamma   An enzyme consisting of cells that contain small granules or rod-shaped structures found in differential staining of the cytoplasm.

DNR   *see* do not resuscitate order

do not resuscitate order (DNR)   Instruction given by a patient or family member not to administer cardiopulmonary resuscitation pending the apparent cessation of life. *See also* living will and no code blue.

Dowdle, Walter R.   Born 1930 in Irvington, Ala., Dowdle received his Ph.D. in microbiology from the University of Maryland in 1960. Since 1970, Director of the Virology Division of the Centers for Disease Control and Prevention and, since 1987, Deputy Director of the Centers for Disease Control and Prevention. Centers for Disease Control and Prevention, 1600 Clifton Road, N.E., Atlanta, GA 30329.

double-blind   A term describing a clinical trial or experimental procedure in which neither the subject nor the researcher knows which treatment (drug or placebo) subjects are receiving.

doxorubicin   A wide-spectrum, antineoplastic, antibiotic agent.

DPT vaccine   A vaccine used for diphtheria, pertussis, and tetanus.

drug abuse   The use or overuse of a drug, generally self-administered, in a manner other than that for which it is prescribed.

drug eruption   Inflammation of the skin characterized by itching, redness, and various skin lesions caused by medication. *Also called* dermatitis medicamentosa.

DSPN   *see* distal symmetric polyneuropathy

Dugas, Gaetan   A French-Canadian flight attendant who was one of the first people in North America to be diagnosed with AIDS.

durable power of attorney   A statement declaring a proxy to administer an individual's wishes concerning medical treatment in the event of incapacity. Durable powers of attorney are not recognized in every state. *See also* medical directive, living will, and no code blue.

dying trajectory   A graphical representation of the dying process. Time is recorded along the horizontal axis and nearness to death along the vertical axis. The condition of the dying individual is plotted across time, with the resulting curve being the dying trajectory.

dyke   *see* lesbian

dysfunction   1) Abnormal, disturbed, impaired, or inadequate functioning of an organ. 2) Abnormal, disturbed, impaired, or inadequate functioning of a social structure, such as a family.

dysphagia   Difficulty in swallowing or the inability to swallow.

dyspnea   Difficult or labored breathing; shortness of breath. Dyspnea is sometimes accompanied by pain.

E

Ebola fever   An acute condition (named for its first known victim in 1976 who came from a village near the Ebola River in Africa) frequently aggravated by hemorrhagic complications and usually fatal.

EBV   *see* Epstein-Barr virus

echocardiography   1) A noninvasive technique for examining the internal structure of the heart. 2) A noninvasive diagnostic method that uses the echoes obtained by directing beams of ultrasonic waves through the chest wall to visualize and graphically record internal cardiac structures. *Also called* ultrasonic cardiography.

ecthyma   An ulcerative inflammation of the skin caused by infection and marked by lesions with crusts or scabs. Variable scarring and pigmentation may result.

edema   A local or generalized condition characterized by excessively large amounts of fluid in the body tissues.

Education and Training Center (ETC)   Any one of a group of geographic-specific sites funded by the Health Resources and Services Administration to provide education to health care professionals about the acquired immunodeficiency syndrome.

EEG   *see* electroencephalogram

efficacy   The power or ability to produce intended effects or results.

EIA   *see* enzyme immunoassay

ejaculation   The expulsion of semen from the male urethra at the peak of sexual excitement.

elderly   1) Past middle age. 2) Aged.

electroencephalogram (EEG)   A recording of the electrical activity of the brain performed by placing electrodes at various locations on the scalp in order to measure the electrical potential. This technique has proven useful as a diagnostic tool in studying convulsive disorders such as epilepsy and in locating cerebral lesions.

electrolyte   1) A substance that yields ions in solution so that its solutions conduct an electric current. 2) Ionized salt in blood, tissue fluids, and cells including chloride, sodium, and potassium.

electrolyte abnormality   A deviation from the normal condition in electrolytes.

elephant leg   *see* elephantiasis

elephantiasis   1) A chronic disease characterized by enlargement of certain body parts (especially the legs and genitals) and by the ulceration and hardening of the surrounding skin. 2) A chronic condition caused by inflammation and obstruction of the lymphatic vessels characterized by pronounced hypertrophy (growth due to increase in size of constituent cells) of the skin and subcutaneous tissues. The disease most frequently effects the lower extremities and scrotum. *Also called* Barbados leg, elephant leg, and pachydermatosis.

ELISA   *see* enzyme-linked immunosorbent assay

encephalitis   Inflammation of the brain.

encephalopathy   Any abnormality of cognitive function.

endemic   Native to a particular population or geographic area.

endocarditis   Inflammation of the lining membrane of the heart (endocardium). It may be due to infection occurring as a primary disorder or may occur in association with another disease. It is usually confined to a heart valve but sometimes affects the lining membrane of the cardiac chambers.

endocrine abnormality   Any deviation in hormonal secretions.

endoscope   An instrument consisting of a tube and optical system for visually examining the inside of a hollow organ or cavity.

endoscopic   Performed by means of an endoscope; pertaining to endoscopy.

endoscopy   Visual inspection of body organs or cavities by means of an endoscope.

enema   1) The injection of solution into the rectum for the purpose of stimulating bowel activity. 2) The introduction of solution for therapeutic or nutritive purposes. 3) The introduction of fluid to aid in roentgenography. 4) A solution introduced into the rectum.

enteric disease   Any pathological condition involving the small intestine.

enteric pathogen   Any microorganism or substance that is capable of producing a disease in the small intestine.

enteritis   Inflammation of the intestine (especially the small intestine).

envelope gene   The gene that encodes the major virion surface envelope glycoprotein (for the human immunodeficiency virus, this glycoprotein is gp160) and is then processed to form a transmembrane segment (gp41) and a glycosylated external segment (gp120). *See also* envelope glycoprotein and glycoprotein.

envelope glycoprotein   The glycosylated external segment (gp120) of the human immunodeficiency virus. The envelope glycoprotein is the major target for the HIV-neutralizing antibody. *See also* glycoprotein.

enzyme immunoassay (EIA)   Any of several methods for measuring the protein and protein-bound molecules concerned with the reaction of an antigen with its specific antibody by using an enzyme covalently linked to an antigen or antibody as a label. The two most common are enzyme-linked immunosorbent assay (ELISA) and enzyme multiplied immunoassay technique (EMIT).

enzyme-linked immunosorbent assay (ELISA)   1) A blood test used to detect the presence of antibodies to the human immunodeficiency virus (HIV). The ELISA is not completely reliable in detecting the presence of HIV antibodies, making it necessary to confirm the results using another test such as the Western blot. 2) Any enzyme immunoassay method in which an enzyme-labeled immunoreactant (antibody or antigen) and an immunosorbent (antibody or antigen bound to a solid support) are used to detect the presence of specific antibodies or antigens. These assays are more sensitive and simple than radioimmune assay tests and do not require the use of radioisotopes and an expensive counting device. *See also* enzyme immunoassay.

eosinophil   A cell, histologic element, or structure readily stained with eosin (a synthetic dye used to stain tissues for microscopic examination). Used especially in reference to a granular leukocyte.

eosinophilic   1) Readily stainable with eosin. 2) Pertaining to eosinophils.

epidemic   The sudden outbreak and rapid spread of an infectious disease among many people within the same geographical area. Also applied to diseases, injuries, or other events that endanger public health. *See also* pandemic.

epidemiology   The science concerned with defining and explaining the interrelationships of the factors determining disease frequency and distribution. Studies are generally undertaken to establish programs for the prevention and control of disease development and spread.

epistaxis   Hemorrhage from the nose; nosebleed.

epithelial cell   An irregularly-shaped cell that has a single nucleus. Frequently, two or three are joined together.

epithelium   The purely cellular, nonvascular layer covering the free surfaces of the body (cutaneous, mucous, and serous).

Epstein-Barr virus (EBV)   A herpes-like virus, discovered in 1964, that is the causative agent in infectious mononucleosis. It is also associated with Burkitt's lymphoma and nasopharyngeal carcinoma.

Erythrocin   *see* erythromycin

erythrocyte   1) A circulating red blood cell. 2) A mature red blood cell or corpuscle shaped in the form of a non-nucleated, yellowish, biconcave disk. It consists of a respiratory pigment (hemoglobin), enclosed in a membrane of proteins and lipoid substances. By the nature of its composition, the erythrocyte is adapted to transport oxygen throughout the body. *Also called* red blood cell or red blood corpuscle.

erythrocyte sedimentation rate (ESR)   The rate at which erythrocytes (the circulating red blood cells) settle from a well-mixed specimen of blood. The ESR is an indicator of inflammatory disease and other conditions in which the rate is usually elevated.

erythrocytophagy   The consumption or engulfment of erythrocytes by other cells (e.g., erythrocytes consumed by histiocytes of the reticuloendothelial system).

erythromycin   An antibiotic produced by Streptomyces erythreus that appears as a yellowish, crystalline powder. Administered orally, it is effective against many gram-positive and certain gram-negative bacteria. It may also be applied topically in the treatment of certain infections. Used to treat patients who are allergic to penicillin and in the treatment of penicillin-resistant infections. The trade name is Erythrocin.

erythrophagocytosis   *see* erythrocytophagy

esophagitis   Inflammation of the esophagus.

esophagoscope   A flexible or rigid instrument, equipped with an optical system, inserted into the esophagus for diagnostic and therapeutic purposes (obtaining specimens or removing foreign substances).

esophagoscopy   An endoscopic examination of the esophagus using an esophagoscope.

Esophotrast   *see* barium sulfate

ESR   *see* erythrocyte sedimentation rate

Essex, Myron   Born 1939 in Coventry, N.J., Essex received his doctorate in veterinary medicine from Michigan State University in 1967 and his Ph.D. in microbiology from the University of California, Davis in 1970. He was one of the early researchers involved in studying the acquired immunodeficiency syndrome. Since 1982 he has been a professor at the School of Public Health and Head of the Department of Cancer Biology, School of Public Health, Harvard University. Department of Microbiology, School of Public Health, Harvard University, 665 Huntington Avenue, Boston, MA 02115.

ETC   *see* Education and Training Center

etiology   The study of the cause or origin of a disease; the cause or origin of a disease.

etoposide   1) An antineoplastic. 2) A semisynthetic derivative of podophyllotoxin, administered intravenously and used to prevent the development, growth, or proliferation of malignant cells.

eustachian dysfunction   Abnormal or impaired functioning of the auditory tube (eustachian tube) that extends from the middle ear to the pharynx. When the passage is blocked, otitis media may develop.

Evatt, Bruce Lee   Born 1939 in Wayne, Okla., Evatt received his M.D. from the University of Oklahoma College of Medicine in 1964. He was one of the first scientists to focus on hemophiliacs and AIDS. Currently an Associate Professor of Medicine at Emory University School of Medicine. Centers for Disease Control and Prevention, 1600 Clifton Road, N.E., Building 1/1407/MS D02, Atlanta, GA 30333, (404) 639-3925.

Expanded Access   A program that allows persons who meet certain criteria but are not enrolled in a clinical trial to receive an experimental drug. The administering physician monitors the person's response to the drug and reports the results to the pharmaceutical company that manufactures the experimental drug.

extrahepatic disease   A pathological condition occurring outside the liver.

F

facial nerve paralysis   Paralysis affecting the muscles of the face in which the seventh cranial nerve is involved.

factor   1) Any substance or activity required to produce a result. 2) A contributing cause in an action. 3) A gene (hereditary factor).

Factor VIII   1) Blood coagulation factor. 2) An antihemophilic factor participating only in the intrinsic pathway of blood coagulation. Deficiency of this factor, when transmitted as a sex-linked recessive trait, causes classic hemophilia. *Also called* antihemophilic globulin (AHG) and antihemophilic factor A.

Fair Housing Amendments Act   Amended numerous times in the 1970s and 1980s, the Act is an outgrowth of the Federal Housing Act of 1968. Designed to ban housing discrimination based on disability and covering most real estate transactions (financing, rental, sale), the Act provides limited exemptions for religious organizations and private clubs, as well as for owners of less than three units who do not use real estate agents and owner-occupied buildings with less than four units.

false negative   1) A test result incorrectly denoting the absence of the abnormality or disease for which the test is administered. 2) An individual whose test result incorrectly excludes him/her from a diagnostic category.

false positive   1) A test result incorrectly denoting the presence of the abnormality or disease for which the test is administered. 2) An individual whose test result incorrectly assigns him/her to a diagnostic category.

Fauci, Anthony   Born 1940 in Brooklyn, N.Y., Fauci received his M.D. from Cornell University Medical College in 1966. He has been the Chief (1980) and Director (1984) of Laboratory Immunoregulation, National Institute of Allergy and Infectious Diseases. In 1988, he became Director of the Office of AIDS Research and Associate Director of the National Institutes of Health, AIDS Research. National Institute of Allergy and Infectious Diseases, National Institutes of Health, Building 31 7A32, Bethesda, MD 20892, (301) 496-2263.

FDA   *see* Food and Drug Administration

feces   1) The excrement, consisting of food residue, bacteria, mucus, and exfoliated cells, discharged from the intestines by way of the anus. 2) Body waste.

Federal Rehabilitation Act   Enacted in 1973, its purpose is to ban discrimination by any federal agency or institution receiving federal financial assistance.

fellatio   Oral stimulation of the penis.

fetus   The unborn offspring of a human or an animal while in the uterus or within an egg during the latter stages of development. In humans, this period is considered to be two to three months after conception until birth. Prior to this period, the fertilized egg is called an embryo.

fever   Elevation of body temperature above normal; hyperpyrexia. The normal body temperature taken orally is 98.6° F. This may vary 1° above or 2° below and still be considered in the normal range. Normal rectal temperatures are 0.5° to 1.0° higher than oral temperatures.

Fischl, Margaret   Born 1950 in New Jersey, Fischl received her M.D. from the University of Miami School of Medicine in 1976. She was one of the principal investigators for AZT. Fischl is currently a full-time academic Associate Professor of Medicine at the University of Miami and is on staff at the Jackson Memorial Hospital in Miami. University of Miami, Department of Medicine, R-60, P.O. Box 016960, Miami, FL 33101, (305) 549-7092.

fist-fucking   *see* brachioproctic eroticism

fisting   *see* brachioproctic eroticism

Fluax   *see* influenza virus vaccine

Fluconazole   An antifungal drug approved by the Food and Drug Administration for the treatment of cryptococcal meningitis and oral and esophogeal candidiasis.

flucytosine   An antifungal drug, appearing as a whitish, crystalline powder, administered orally to treat yeast and fungal infections (including those caused by Candida and/or Cryptococcus such as endocarditis, septicemia, and urinary tract infections). The trade name is Ancobon.

Fluogen   *see* influenza virus vaccine

folic acid   A member of the vitamin B complex necessary for various metabolic reactions and used in the treatment of sprue. Inadequate amounts of folic acid cause megaloblastic anemia. Folic acid is found naturally in green plants, liver, and yeast. *Also called* Lactobacillus casei factor, liver Lactobacillus casei factor, pteroylglutamic acid, and vitamin M. The trade name is Folvite.

folinic acid   A derivative of folic acid used to counteract the effects of folic acid antagonists and to treat anemia caused by a deficiency of folic acid. *Also called* citrovorum factor and leucovorin. The trade name is Calcium Folinate.

follicle   A small sac or cavity for excretion or secretion.

folliculitis   Inflammation of a follicle or follicles.

Folvite   *see* folic acid

Food and Drug Administration (FDA)   Founded in 1931 under the Agriculture Appropriation Act, it is charged with protecting the U.S. population against impure and unsafe foods, cosmetics, drugs, and other potential hazards. Food and Drug Administration, Department of Health and Human Services, Public Health Service, 5600 Fishers Lane, Rockville, MD 20857.

Foscarnet   *see* phosphonoformate

Foundation of Pharmacists and Corporate America for AIDS Education Founded in 1988, this organization consists of associations, corporations, pharmacies, and individuals that seek to support pharmacists who provide education and outreach programs designed to prevent the spread of HIV and AIDS. It is located at 700 Fifth Street, N.W., Suite 303, Washington, DC 20001, (202) 371-1830.

Four H Club A slang term applied by American epidemiologists in the early years of the epidemic to describe the populations most severely affected by it. The term referred to Haitians, homosexuals, heroin addicts, and hemophiliacs (and, in some cases, hookers). It is now considered inappropriate because it perpetuates the stigmatization associated with HIV and AIDS.

Francis, Donald Pinkston Born 1942 in Los Angeles, Francis received his M.D. from Northwestern University in 1968. He has been Chief of the Epidemiology Branch, Hepatitis Laboratories Division, Centers for Disease Control and Prevention, since 1978. Francis was one of the first members of the CDC to believe that a new sexually transmitted disease was causing immune deficiencies in homosexual men. Center for Infectious Diseases, Centers for Disease Control and Prevention, 1600 Clifton Road, N.E., Atlanta, GA 30333.

free base A form of cocaine in which the hydrochloride salt is alkalinized, extracted with an organic solvent (e.g., ether), and then heated. After inhalation, the drug is absorbed rapidly through the lungs.

freebasing The inhalation of a form of cocaine known as free base.

French kiss 1) A passionate kiss with the lips parted and tongues touching. 2) To kiss passionately with the lips parted and tongues touching.

Friedman-Kein, Alvin Emanuel Born 1934 in New York City, Friedman-Kein received his M.D. from Yale University School of Medicine in 1960. Currently a Professor in the Department of Dermatology and Microbiology at New York University, he is also on staff at NYU Medical Center and Goldwater Memorial Hospital in New York City. Friedman-Kein was one of the first to describe the outbreak of Kaposi's sarcoma among gay males in New York at the outset of the epidemic. Office address: 530 First Avenue, New York, NY 10016, (212) 340-7380.

fungal encephalitis   Inflammation of the brain resulting from invasion by a pathogenic fungus.

fungal infection   The state or condition in which the body, or a part of it, is invaded by a pathogenic fungus.

fungi   Plural of fungus.

fungicidin   *see* nystatin

fungus   A general term used to denote a group of vegetable cellular organisms that are characterized by the absence of chlorophyll. They exist on organic matter and are generally simple in structure and form. Included in this group are molds, yeasts, rusts, and mushrooms.

furuncle   A painful, deep-seated nodule formed in the skin by circumscribed inflammation, enclosing a central core. It is caused by staphylococci, which enter through the hair follicles. Formation is promoted by local irritation and digestive derangement. It usually ends in pus formation and necrosis. *Also called* boil and furunculus.

furunculosis   The   persistent   simultaneous   occurrence   of furuncles.

furunculus   *see* furuncle

G

gag gene   The gene that encodes the major internal viral structural proteins of the human immunodeficiency virus (p17, p24, p15).

Gallo, Robert C.   Born 1937 in Waterbury, Conn., Gallo received his M.D. from Jefferson Medical College in 1963. Since 1972, Director of the National Cancer Institute. National Cancer Institute, NIH Building 37, Room #6A-09, Bethesda, MD 20892.

ganciclovir   1) A drug used to treat cytomegalovirus retinitis. 2) An acyclic nucleoside structurally related to acyclovir and an effective antiviral against cytomegalovirus in vitro. The drug has been carefully studied only in the treatment of cytomegalovirus retinitis and has been shown to halt retinal destruction during administration. When administration is withdrawn, disease progression resumes. Licensed by the Food and Drug Administration in 1989 for treating sight-threatening cytomegalovirus retinitis, its use for treatment of other CMV diseases is still considered investigational.

ganglion   1) A collection of nerve cell bodies located outside the central nervous system. 2) A benign cystic tumor developing on a tendon or aponeurosis, sometimes occurring in the back of the wrist or dorsum of the foot. 3) A knot-like mass.

gastric anacidity   *see* achlorhydria

gastrointestinal dysfunction   Abnormal, impaired, or inadequate functioning of the stomach and intestines.

gastrointestinal tract   The stomach and intestines.

gay   Homosexual. Generally refers to male homosexuals, but may also include homosexual women. The term has political, psychological, and social implications that go beyond the realm of sexual orientation. *See also* homosexual and lesbian.

gay bowel syndrome   A general term used to denote a constellation of intestinal diseases among gay men including proctitis, proctocolitis, and enteritis. The term was widely used in the 1970's with the dramatic increase in enteric diseases within the gay community thought to be directly linked to anal intercourse.

gay lymph-node syndrome   A term applied to generalized lymphadenopathy (with benign reactive changes shown in biopsy) prior to 1981 when the Centers for Disease Control and Prevention published the first description of persistent generalized lymphadenopathy.

Gay Men's Health Crisis (GMHC)   Founded in 1982 as a social service agency for the clinical treatment of the acquired immunodeficiency syndrome, GMHC provides a variety of services (therapy, education, recreation services, crisis counseling, a buddy program, and advocacy) to AIDS patients and their families. GMHC also maintains a hotline, speakers' bureau and library, sponsors AIDS education programs, and compiles statistics. Gay Men's Health Crisis, 129 W. 20th Street, New York, NY 10011, (212) 337-3519.

gay plague   Since gay men were the first infected and continue to constitute the greatest number of reported cases in the United States, this term was often used to denote the acquired immunodeficiency syndrome, particularly in the early years of the epidemic.

gay pneumonia   Term used in the early years of the epidemic to denote Pneumocystis carinii pneumonia.

gay-related immune deficiency (GRID)   One of a group of names initially used to denote the acquired immunodeficiency syndrome. The current name was adopted in 1981. *See also* acquired community immune deficiency syndrome, community acquired immune deficiency syndrome, and acquired immunodeficiency syndrome.

gene   The basic biological unit of heredity. They are self-producing, ultramicroscopic structures that are transmitted from parent to offspring. Each gene is a segment on a DNA molecule that stores the information necessary for the transcription of information by RNA and synthesis of proteins and occupies a specific location on a chromo-some. Hereditary traits are dependent on the pairing of genes in the same position on a pair of chromosomes.

genetic research   The study and examination of reproduction, heredity, and its variance.

genital wart   1) A small tumorous growth on the skin of the genitalia caused by a virus. 2) A circumscribed epidermal lesion of the genitalia with a horny surface caused by a human papillomavirus.

genitalia   The various internal and external organs concerned with reproduction.

genus   In biology, the taxonomic division between the species and the family.

Giardia   A genus of flagellate protozoa, usually nonpathogenic. They inhabit the small intestine in humans and are characterized by the presence of a large sucking disk on the ventral body surface (the means by which the organism attaches itself to the intestinal epithelium).

Giardia intestinalis   *see* Giardia lamblia

Giardia lamblia   A species of Giardia found in humans that may cause giardiasis. They are transmitted by ingestion of fecally con-taminated matter and are found worldwide. *Also called* Giardia intestinalis and Lamblia intestinalis.

giardiasis   1) A protozoan infection. 2) A common infection with the flagellate protozoan Giardia lamblia. Infection is spread through contaminated food or water. Most cases are asymptomatic. When present, symptoms include anorexia, cramps, diarrhea, fever, nau-sea, weakness, weight loss, and vomiting. *Also called* lambliasis.

GLQ-223   A drug derived from the Chinese cucumber tested in Phase I clinical trials and shown to be effective against the human immunodeficiency virus in vitro by selectively destroying infected cells. The drug is now being tested in Phase II trials.

glutathione   1) A combination of amino acids fundamentally im-portant in cellular respiration; takes up and gives off hydrogen. 2) A tripeptide of glutamate, cysteine, and glycine found in small quantities in active animal and plant tissues. It is essential for cellular respiration and functions in redox reactions such as serving as a cofactor for enzymes and destroying or detoxifying harmful compounds.

glycoprotein   1) Any of a class of compounds in which a carbohydrate group is combined with a protein. 2) Any of a class of compounds (this group includes the mucins, the mucoids, and the chondroproteins) consisting of a carbohydrate and a protein. In decomposition, they yield a product frequently capable of reducing alkaline solutions of cupric oxide.

GMHC   *see* Gay Men's Health Crisis

Goedert, James Jerome   Born 1951, Goedert received his M.D. from Loyola University of Chicago, Stritch School of Medicine, Maywood, Ill. He was one of the first to link AIDS to homosexual males and originally promoted the theory of nitrite inhalant as a causative agent for the acquired immunodeficiency syndrome. Office address: 3C-19 Landon, Bethesda, MD 20817.

golden shower   The act of urinating on an individual (or being urinated on) for sexual pleasure. *See also* water sport.

gonad   1) A gland or organ that produces reproductive cells in animals. 2) A general term referring to a gamete-producing gland; it includes both the female ovary and male testis.

gonorrhea   1) An infectious venereal disease. 2) A specific contagious inflammation of the genital mucous membrane of either sex caused by infection due to Neisseria gonorrhoeae. Often asymptomatic in females, gonorrhea is characterized by urethritis in males and accompanied by slow, painful urination containing mucus and pus. Other parts of the body (heart, throat, joints, rectum, and skin) may also be affected.

gossypol   A toxic chemical (with antifertility properties in males) that is yellowish in appearance and found in cotton seed. It is detoxified by heating.

Gottlieb, Michael Stuart   Born 1947 in New Brunswick, N.J., Gottlieb received his M.D. from the University of Rochester in 1973.

Since 1980, an Assistant Professor of Medicine at the School of Medicine, University of California, Los Angeles. Gottlieb was the founder of the National AIDS Research Foundation, which merged with the AIDS Medical Foundation to form the American Foundation for AIDS Research. Office address: 1260 15th Street, Suite 808, Santa Monica, CA 90404.

gp41   The transmembrane segment of the human immunodeficiency virus.

gp120   The glycosylated external segment of the human immunodeficiency virus (envelope glycoprotein).

gp160   1) The envelope gene of the human immunodeficiency virus. 2) A precursor polypeptide that is glycosylated and cleaved to yield gp120.

gram-negative bacteria   Bacteria that, in Gram's method of staining, lose the stain and take the color of the red counterstain.

gram-positive bacteria   Bacteria that, in Gram's method of staining, retain the stain.

Gram's method   A differential method of staining bacteria for classification purposes in which the specimen is first placed in aniline water-gentian violet or carbolic gentian violet, rinsed in water, and immersed in an iodine solution, rinsed in water again and placed in strong alcohol for several minutes, rinsed again, and dipped in a dilute eosin solution. Gram-negative bacteria decolorize and assume the counterstain, while gram-positive bacteria stain a dark violet. This artificial coloring of bacteria is used to facilitate examination under the microscope.

GRID   *see* gay-related immune deficiency

Grieco, Michael H.   Grieco received his M.D. from Columbia University in 1979. Since 1973, Chief of the Division of Allergy, Clinical Immunology, and Infectious Diseases at St. Luke's-Roosevelt Hospital Center in New York. He was a major researcher on AZT. Department of Clinical Medicine, Columbia University, 630 W. 168th Street, New York, NY 10032.

grief The normal emotional response to a recognized loss. A process through which the bereaved pass in order to recover from the loss; it produces both emotional and physical manifestations.

group-specific complement Any of a series of enzymatic proteins in normal serum that, in the presence of a sensitizer specific for a given group, destroy bacteria and other cells. The complement is important in maintaining a normal state of health. *See also* immunity, antibody, and antigen.

guerilla clinic Any of a group of for-profit facilities established early in the AIDS epidemic for the purpose of dispensing black-market drugs or providing treatments or therapies not approved in traditional medical channels.

Guinan, Mary Elizabeth Born 1939 in New York City, Guinan received her Ph.D. in physiology from the University of Texas, Medical Branch, Galveston, in 1969 and her M.D. from Johns Hopkins University in 1972. Since 1978, Clinical Research Investigator of Venereal Diseases, Centers for Disease Control and Prevention. She was one of the original members of a CDC task force established to investigate the outbreak of Kaposi's sarcoma and Pneumocystis carinii pneumonia in the homosexual community at the outset of the epidemic. Centers for Disease Control and Prevention, 1600 Clifton Road, N.E., Atlanta, GA 30333.

gummatous syphilis Late benign syphilis.

gynecological disorder A disturbance in any of the female reproductive organs, including the breasts.

Gyne-Lotrimin *see* clotrimazole

H

hairy leukoplakia (HL)   A white lesion generally found on the lateral margins of the tongue. Lesions may vary in size and shape and have an irregular surface. They may spread to cover the dorsal surface of the tongue and downwards on to the ventral surface. Hairy leukoplakia is usually asymptomatic and is most likely viral induced (Epstein-Barr virus has been associated with HL tissue).

Haitian Coalition on AIDS (HCA)   Founded in 1983, this organization is divided into local, state, and regional groups. It seeks to educate the general public about AIDS and its effect on the Haitian community, promote AIDS education to the Haitian community, and provide services to those members of the community with AIDS and their families. Haitian Coalition on AIDS, 50 Court Street, Suite 605, Brooklyn, NY 11201, (718) 855-0972.

half-life   The amount of time required for one-half of a substance to be eliminated from the living tissue, organ, or organism into which it has been introduced.

Hassal's corpuscles   Oval or spherical bodies present in the medulla of the thymus consisting of concentrically arranged epithelial cells surrounding a core of degenerated cells.

HBV   *see* hepatitis B virus

HCA   *see* Haitian Coalition on AIDS

HCW   *see* health care worker

health care   The charge of providing for mental and physical well-being.

Health Care Financing Administration   Established in 1977, it is a principal operating component of the Department of Health and Human Services. The Administration oversees Medicare and Medicaid Programs and related federal medical care quality-control staffs. Health Care Financing Administration, Department of Health and Human Services, 200 Independence Avenue, S.W., Washington, DC 20201, (202) 245-6113.

health care provider   An individual who furnishes the means by which others obtain mental and physical well-being (e.g., physicians, nurses).

health care worker (HCW)   An individual who is employed in the profession responsible for the provision of mental and physical well-being (e.g., medical professionals, laboratory personnel, technicians, physical facility staff).

Health Resources and Services Administration (HRSA)   The administration responsible for leadership within the Public Health Service concerning general health services and resource issues relating to access, cost, equity, and quality of care. It funds service demonstration projects in major cities, establishes centers to train health care professionals about AIDS, supports renovation of health care facilities for AIDS patients, and awards pediatric health care grants for the care of babies with AIDS. Health Resources and Services Administration, Department of Health and Human Services, Public Health Service, 5600 Fishers Lane, Rockville, MD 20857.

helminthic infestation   Invasion by and harboring of parasitic worms that produce injurious effects.

helper cell   Differentiated T lymphocyte whose cooperation is necessary for the production of antibodies against most antigens. Helper cells are marked by the T4 antigen in humans. *See also* lymphocyte.

hematologic abnormality   A deviation from the norm in the blood or blood-forming tissues.

hemodialysis   A method for artificially performing the function of the kidneys (in removing wastes or toxins from the blood) by circulating the blood through a series of tubes made of semipermeable membranes that are bathed in solutions that selectively remove undesirable elements.

hemodialyzer   An apparatus used in performing hemodialysis.

hemoglobin   1) The oxygen-carrying pigment of the red blood cells. 2) The iron-containing pigment of the erythrocytes. It is formed by the developing erythrocyte in bone marrow and serves to transport oxygen from the lungs to the tissues.

hemophilia   A hereditary blood disease characterized by prolonged coagulation time. The blood fails to clot and hemorrhage occurs. Although transmitted by the female who carries the recessive gene, hemophilia occurs almost exclusively in males. There are two main forms: hemophilia A (classic hemophilia), resulting from factor VIII deficiency, and hemophilia B, resulting from factor IX deficiency.

hemophiliac   An individual exhibiting hemophilia.

hemorrhage   The abnormal discharge of blood from the vessels. It may be arterial, capillary, or venous from blood vessels into tissues or into or from the body. Hemorrhages are classified according to size, with very small as petechiae, up to 1 centimeter as purpura, and larger as ecchymoses.

hemorrhagic   Pertaining to or characterized by hemorrhage.

hepatitis   Inflammation of the liver caused by bacterial invasion, chemical or physical agents, or viral infections; generally characterized by an enlarged liver, fever, and jaundice accompanied by abnormalities of liver function.

hepatitis B   A viral disease caused by the hepatitis B virus. It is endemic worldwide and transmitted primarily by parenteral routes (e.g., blood transfusions, sharing of needles), intimate personal contact (e.g., sexual contact), and perinatally from mother to fetus. In the initial stage, there may be anorexia, fever, malaise, nausea, and vomiting. These decline with the onset of clinical jaundice, arthritis, and angioedema.

hepatitis B virus (HBV)   An unclassified DNA virus having complex, double-layered virions, a double-stranded genome, and three major antigens (the hepatitis B core antigen, surface antigen, and e antigen). It is the causative agent of hepatitis B.

hepatobiliary symptoms   Any perceptive change in the liver, bile, or biliary ducts indicating disease.

hepatomegaly   Enlargement of the liver.

heroin   *see* diacetylmorphine

herpes encephalitis   Encephalitis due to infection with herpesvirus.

herpes simplex   An acute infectious disease caused by herpes simplex virus type 1 or 2. It is characterized by the development of one or more small, fluid-filled, thin-walled vesicles occurring as a primary infection or recurring because of reactivation of a latent infection. Type 1 infections generally do not involve genital areas of the body, whereas type 2 infections do. Acyclovir applied locally has been an effective form of treatment, with antibiotics often used to treat secondary infections.

herpes zoster   An acute infectious disease caused by the varicella-zoster virus. It is characterized by inflammation of the sensory ganglia. Severe neuralgic pain and vesicular eruption occur along the affected nerve. It is generally unilateral and is self-limited. It is believed that herpes zoster represents reactivation of latent varicella-zoster virus in individuals who previously presented with chicken pox and were rendered partially immune. Shingles is synonymous with herpes zoster.

herpesvirus   Any one of a large group of DNA viruses important in humans and found in many animal species. The viruses mature in the nucleus of the infected cell, where they cause the formation of a characteristic inclusion body (some also cause the formation of a cytoplasmic inclusion body). Included in this group are herpes simplex virus type 1, herpes simplex virus type 2, cytomegalovirus, and Epstein-Barr virus.

heterosexual   1) An individual whose sexual orientation is to people of the opposite sex. 2) Pertaining to the opposite sex. 3) The opposite of homosexual. *Also called* straight.

heterosexuality   Sexual attraction toward a person or persons of the opposite sex.

Hirsch, Martin Stanley   Born 1939 in Cortland, N.Y., Hirsch received his M.D. from Johns Hopkins University in 1964. Since 1988, he has been a Professor in the Department of Medicine, Harvard Medical School. Hirsch was one of the principal investigators for AZT. Massachusetts General Hospital, Department of Medicine, Harvard Medical School, Boston, MA 02114.

histopathology   The study of the microscopic structure of diseased tissues.

Histoplasma capsulatum   The causative agent of histoplasmosis, which grows as a fungus and as a yeast and occurs as small, oval, yeast-like cells in tissue that appear to be encapsulated but are not.

histoplasmosis   A respiratory disease due to the inhalation of Histoplasma capsulatum. Infection is generally asymptomatic. When symptoms appear, they range from a mild self-limited infection to severe illness (anemia, fever, acute pneumonia, leukopenia, enlargement of the spleen and liver, and gastrointestinal ulcers). It may be treated by administering amphotericin B intravenously.

history-taking   Systematically recording past events as they relate to a person or group of people.

HIV   *see* human immunodeficiency virus

HIV encephalitis   *see* AIDS dementia complex

HIV encephalopathy   *see* AIDS dementia complex

HIV-1   *see* human immunodeficiency virus type 1

HIV-2   *see* human immunodeficiency virus type 2

HIVID   *see* dideoxycytidine

HIV wasting syndrome   The loss of weight and strength often accompanying infection with the human immunodeficiency virus that results in emaciation and enfeeblement. *Also called* slim disease and wasting syndrome.

HL   *see* hairy leukoplakia

HLA   *see* human leukocyte antigen

Ho, David D.   Born 1952, Ho received his M.D. from Harvard Medical School in 1978. Director of the Aaron Diamond AIDS Research Center. Aaron Diamond AIDS Research Center, c/o Aaron Diamond Foundation, 1270 Avenue of the Americas, Suite 2624, New York, NY 10020, (212) 767-7680.

Hodgkin's disease   A form of malignant lymphoma of unknown cause characterized by painless, progressive enlargement of the lymph nodes, lymphoid tissue, liver, and spleen. Other symptoms may include anemia, anorexia, fever, night sweats, severe itching, and weight loss. It may appear as acute, localized, latent with relapsing fever, lymphogranulomatosis, and splenomegaly.

home care   The provision of health care in a patient's home. *Also called* home health care.

home health care   *see* home care

homosexual   1) An individual whose sexual orientation is toward persons of the same sex. 2) Pertaining to the same sex. 3) The opposite of heterosexual. *Also called* gay.

homosexuality   Sexual attraction toward a person or persons of the same sex.

hooker   *see* prostitute

hospice   1) An interdisciplinary approach to providing palliative and supportive care (economic, physical, social, and spiritual services) for the terminally ill. These services may be administered in a patient's home or in a hospice facility. 2) A facility that provides palliative and supportive services for the terminally ill.

host   The organism (plant or animal) that harbors or nourishes a parasite.

Hoth, Daniel Floyd, Jr.   Born 1946, Hoth received his M.D. from Georgetown University in 1972. He was recruited to administer the AIDS Clinical Trails Group when the early AIDS program faltered. National Cancer Institute, 4C09, Bethesda, MD 20892.

hotline   Telephone service providing crisis intervention to individuals experiencing severe problems (alcoholism, child abuse, spousal abuse, suicide, rape, etc.). It is usually staffed continuously by paraprofessionals or professionals in the medical or social sciences. In the HIV/AIDS arena, hotlines also typically provide answers to questions about the disease and offer referrals to local service providers.

HPA-23   *see* antimoniotungstate

HPV   *see* human papillomavirus

HRSA   *see* Health Resources and Services Administration

HTLV   *see* human T-cell lymphotrophic virus

HTLV-III   *see* human immunodeficiency virus

human immunodeficiency virus (HIV)   The virus that causes acquired immunodeficiency syndrome (AIDS). It is a retrovirus that infects the T4 lymphocyte cells, monocyte-macrophage cells, certain cell populations in the brain and spinal cord, and colorectal epithelial cells. HIV-infected cells weaken the immune system. Individuals infected with the human immunodeficiency virus do not necessarily have AIDS. Previously called lymphadenopathy virus, human T-cell leukemia virus III, and human T-cell lymphotrophic virus III. *See also* acquired immunodeficiency syndrome.

human immunodeficiency virus type 1 (HIV-1)   One of two main classes of the human immunodeficiency virus, considered to be more virulent than type 2. In the United States, this is the most common form.

human immunodeficiency virus type 2 (HIV-2)   One of two main classes of the human immunodeficiency virus, considered to be less virulent than type 1. Discovered in West Africa, it does not appear to be as prevalent in the United States as HIV-1.

human leukocyte antigen (HLA)   The histocompatibility antigen governed by genes of the major human complex that controls the ability of cells to survive without immunological interference.

human papillomavirus (HPV)   A subgroup of the papovaviruses causing papillomas or warts. *See also* papovavirus.

human T-cell leukemia virus   *see* human T-cell lymphotrophic virus

human T-cell leukemia virus III (HTLV-III)   *see* human immunodeficiency virus

human T-cell lymphotrophic virus (HTLV)   A family of retroviruses that are lymphocytotrophic and particularly partial to T lymphocytes of the inducer/helper subset. *Also called* human T-cell leukemia virus.

humoral abnormality   A deformity or deviation from the norm in body fluids (the antibody limb of protection).

humoral immunity   Immunity that is accomplished by the aid of antibodies.

hydrocortisone   The corticosteroid hormone produced by the human adrenal cortex and produced synthetically. It is essential in maintaining life, sustaining blood pressure, and providing mineralocorticoid activity. Used in the treatment of various ailments (e.g., allergies, collagen abnormalities, inflammations, and certain neoplasms).

hypercapnia   An excess of carbon dioxide in the blood.

hyperglycemia   An increased amount of sugar in the blood resulting in a condition that may lower resistance to infection and may precede diabetic coma.

hyperkalemia (also hyperkaliemia)   An increased amount of potassium in the blood generally caused by defective renal excretion.

hyperplasia   An abnormal increase in the number of normal cells in the normal tissue arrangement.

hypertension   A condition in which the patient has persistently high arterial blood pressure. The cause of hypertension may be unknown, or associated with the presence of other diseases.

hyperthermia   1) Unusually high body temperature. 2) Therapy in which the body temperature is raised to an abnormal height to treat disease.

hypertrophy   The enlargement or growth of an organ or structure (not involving tumor formation) due to an increase in the size of its constituent cells.

hypodermic   Administered or inserted under the skin. Hypodermic administration/insertion is used when a drug cannot be administered orally, readily absorbed in the gastrointestinal tract, or when gastrointestinal secretions would alter the drug. It may also be used to provide local anesthesia to the site of injection.

hypoglycemia   A decreased amount of sugar in the blood. This condition may result in shakiness, cold sweat, fatigue, hypothermia, headache, and malaise, accompanied by confusion, irritability, and weakness. Hypoglycemia may ultimately result in seizures, coma, and possibly death.

hypogonadism   A condition involving decreased functional activity and secretion of the gonads, resulting in slowed growth and sexual development or, in the adult, impairment of normal sexual function.

hypokalemia   A decreased amount of potassium in the circulating blood. It may result from a loss of potassium through renal secretion or through expulsion via the gastrointestinal tract (i.e., diarrhea or vomiting). Hypokalemia may be manifested by muscular weakness and paralysis, postural hypotension, renal disease, and gastrointestinal dysfunction.

hyponatremia   A decreased amount of sodium in the blood.

hypopharynx   The lowermost division of the pharynx, which lies below the epiglottis and leads to the larynx and esophagus.

hypotension   A decrease in blood pressure below normal. It may be caused by dehydration, shock, fever, anemia, cancer, and various diseases that result in debilitation or wasting and impending death.

hypothermia   Having a body temperature that is below normal. This may be due to prolonged exposure to extreme cold or may be induced artificially. Hypothermia is induced to lower the rate of metabolism, thereby reducing oxygen need. Used in various surgical procedures, especially cardiovascular and neurological procedures.

hypovolemia   A decreased volume of blood in the body.

hypoxemia   Deficient oxygenation of the blood. *See also* hypoxia.

hypoxia   1) A decreased amount of oxygen. 2) A decreased concentration of oxygen in the blood distributed to tissue.

I

ibuprofen 1) A common anti-inflammatory available with or without a prescription. 2) A non-steroidal anti-inflammatory agent used in the treatment of osteoarthritis and rheumatoid arthritis. Trade names are Advil, Motrin, and Nuprin.

ichthyosis A noninflammatory condition in which the skin is dry and scaly. Depending on the stage and degree of the condition, it has been described in terms of various animals (i.e., as alligator skin, crocodile skin, or fish skin).

icterus *see* jaundice

ICU *see* intensive care unit

idiopathic inflammatory pulmonary disease A pathologic condition of unknown origin causing inflammation of the lungs. It is not a result of any other disease.

idiopathic thrombocytopenic purpura (ITP) A form of a purpura often accompanied by the presence of a serum antiplatelet antibody, unassociated with any definable systemic disease in which the blood platelet count is decreased.

IL-1 *see* interleukin-1

IL-2 *see* interleukin-2

immune system A complex system made up of various cellular and molecular components that defends the body against foreign substances. Lymphocytes and macrophages are the primary cellular components, and antibodies and lymphokines are the primary molecular components. Granulocytes and the complement system are involved in immune responses but are not necessarily considered part of the immune system.

immune system abnormality   A deviation in the normal functioning of the immune system.

immune thrombocytopenic purpura   A form of purpura occurring as a consequence of a disturbance in the immune system (e.g., infection with the human immunodeficiency virus) in which the platelet count is decreased.

immunity   1) The state or condition of being protected from a disease, especially an infectious one. It is usually induced by immunization, previous infection, or by other nonimmunologic factors. 2) The response of the body and its tissues to a variety of antigens, including pollens, red cells, transplanted tissues, or the individual's own cells.

immunization   1) Becoming immune. 2) Inducing immunity; rendering a patient immune.

immunodeficiency   Compromised or decreased ability to respond to antigenic stimuli (i.e., to resist disease agents). It is classified as antibody, cellular, combined deficiency, or phagocytic dysfunction disorders. *See also* acquired immunodeficiency syndrome.

immunology   The branch of science dealing with the study of immunity.

immunopathogenesis   A process in which the course of a disease is affected/altered by an immune response or by the products of an immune response.

immunosuppression   The prevention or diminution of the formation of immune response.

impetigo   A contagious, inflammatory skin disease caused by direct inoculation of group A streptococci or Staphylococcus aureus into superficial cutaneous abrasions or compromised skin. It is marked by isolated pustules that rupture to discharge an amber-colored fluid composed of serum and pus that dries to form a thick, yellowish crust. The pustules may spread peripherally but are usually found around the nose and mouth.

impotence   1) The inability of the male to achieve or maintain penile erection. 2) Weakness.

Imreg   A natural, leukocyte-derived, polypeptide immunomodulator that has been shown to enhance production of certain lymphokines in the laboratory.

Imuran   *see* azathioprine

imuthiol   An organic compound that contains sulfur and is an inducer of T lymphocytes. It has been shown to have anti-HIV activity in vitro.

in vitro   In an artificial environment, outside the living body.

in vitro cultivation   The propagation of living organisms in an artificial environment such as a Petri dish or test tube.

in vivo   Within the living body; in a living organism.

inactivation agent   An agent used to destroy biological activity, as of an enzyme, microorganism, or virus (e.g., heat).

INAPEN   *see* International AIDS Prospective Epidemiology Network

incidence   1) The rate of new occurrence of any event over a period of time in relation to the population within which it occurs (e.g., the number of new cases of a disease). 2) The act or manner of falling upon or influencing.

incontinence   1) The inability to control excretory functions (e.g., defecation, urination). 2) The absence of restraint; immoderation or excess.

incubation   1) The interval between exposure to a pathogen and the appearance of the first clinical symptom in the development of an infectious disease. 2) The development of bacteria culture under controlled conditions. 3) The development of a fertilized egg. 4) The care of a premature infant in a controlled environment to promote development and survival.

incubation period   The latent interval during which an infection or disease is present without manifesting itself.

IND   *see* Investigational New Drug

index case   The initial individual whose state of health prompted investigation into a disorder.

Index Medicus   *see* Cumulated Index Medicus

Individual Treatment IND   A program established by the Food and Drug Administration in which a person may receive an experimental drug free of charge from the pharmaceutical manufacturer with the assistance of a personal physician. Admission to this program is granted on an individual basis by the FDA. *See also* Investigational New Drug.

induced immunosuppression   The prevention or diminution of an immune response by artificial means.

indurate   1) To harden. 2) Hardened.

infant   A liveborn child from birth through one year of age. *See also* neonate.

infection   The state or condition in which the body or part of it is invaded by microorganisms. The microorganisms will multiply under conditions favorable to them, producing injurious results. If the body's defense mechanisms are effective, the infection will remain localized. If the body's defense mechanisms are not capable of staving off the invasion and multiplication, the local infection may persist and spread.

infectious agent   1) Something that produces infection. 2) Something that is capable of being transmitted with or without contact.

infectious mononucleosis   An acute infectious disease that primarily affects lymphoid tissue and is characterized by enlarged lymph nodes and spleen with an increase in abnormal mononuclear leukocytes in the blood. It is associated with Epstein-Barr virus.

inflammatory bowel disease   A general term used to denote those inflammatory diseases of the bowel of unknown origin (e.g., ulcerative colitis, Crohn's disease, regional enteritis).

inflammatory neuropathy   Inflammation of the peripheral nervous system causing abnormal function.

influenza virus vaccine   A sterile suspension of killed influenza virus types A and B, either individually or combined. Commonly known as a "flu shot." Trade names are Fluax and Fluogen.

informed consent   Permission voluntarily granted for any medical procedure, test, or medication by a competent individual. It is based on an understanding of the alternatives, nature, risks, and possible benefits involved.

insertive anal intercourse   Sexual intercourse in which the individual inserts the penis into the anus of his partner. *Also called* active anal intercourse.

intensive care   Service provided by skilled medical personnel to seriously ill patients requiring special equipment and continuous attention. It is usually provided in a designated area of the care facility (i.e., an intensive care unit).

intensive care unit (ICU)   A designated area within the care facility that provides special equipment and continuous attention by medical personnel to the seriously ill.

intercourse   Interaction between individuals or groups. *See also* sexual intercourse, homosexual sexual intercourse, anal intercourse, insertive anal intercourse, receptive anal intercourse, and vaginal intercourse.

interferon   Any of the glycoproteins that are formed when cells are exposed to viral or other foreign nucleic acids and that exert host-specific but not viral-specific antiviral activities. Interferons are important in immune function, have antitumor activity, and can repress the growth of nonviral parasites within the cells. *See also* alpha interferon.

interleukin-1 (IL-1)   A substance produced by macrophages that induces the production of interleukin-2 by T cells that have been stimulated by antigen or mitogen.

interleukin-2 (IL-2)   1) An anticancer drug; its side effects are sometimes fatal. 2) A lymphokine produced by T cells in response to antigenic or mitogenic stimulation and the signal carried by interleukin-1. It stimulates the growth and proliferation of T lymphocytes.

International AIDS Prospective Epidemiology Network (INAPEN)   Founded in 1984, this organization seeks to heighten the effectiveness of research in the AIDS arena by promoting cooperation, data sharing, and standardization of research methodologies. In addition to fostering collaborative research, it maintains a biographical archives and compiles statistics to aid in research. International AIDS Prospective Epidemiology Network, 155 N. Harbor Drive, No. 5103, Chicago, IL 60601, (312) 565-2109.

intertriginous infection   1) Inflammation occurring in the folds of the skin. 2) A superficial dermatitis occurring in the folds of the skin such as the creases in the neck, between the toes, or the groin. It is characterized by redness, maceration, burning, itching, and occasionally ulceration and erosion.

intertrigo labialis   *see* perleche

intracranial disorder   Any pathological condition situated within the skull.

intrahepatic disease   Any pathological condition within the liver that produces a group of clinical symptoms peculiar to it and that sets it apart as abnormal.

intrapartum   Occurring during childbirth or delivery.

intrathecal   1) Within the spinal cord. 2) Within a sheath.

intrathoracic adenopathy   Swelling of the gland or lymph nodes within the chest.

intravenous (IV)   Within or into a vein or veins.

intravenous drug abuser (IVDA)   *see* intravenous drug user

intravenous drug user (IVDU)   An individual who uses or overuses any drug that is injected into a vein in a manner that deviates from the drug's intended use. *Also called* intravenous drug abuser (IVDA).

intubation   The insertion of a tube into a body canal or into any hollow organ (e.g., the trachea, to permit the entrance of air).

invasive nutritional substitute   Any nutrient administered intravenously.

invasive procedure   A technique involving the puncture of the skin or the insertion of foreign matter by using a device, needle, or tube to enter the body.

Investigational New Drug (IND)   The status provided by the Food and Drug Administration that allows a compound to be tested on humans for the first time. *See also* Individual Treatment IND.

iodoquinol   An antiamebic agent appearing as a yellowish to tan crystalline powder used in the treatment of amebiasis and Trichomonas hominis infection of the intestine and Trichomonas vaginalis vaginitis. It is administered orally in the treatment of intestinal disorders and intravaginally for vaginitis. *Also called* diiodohydroxyquin. The trade name is Yodoxin.

IPV   *see* poliovirus vaccine inactivated

ischemia   Local deficiency of blood supply due to functional constriction or actual obstruction of a blood vessel.

ischemic   Pertaining to or affected with ischemia.

isoniazid   An odorless antibacterial compound appearing as colorless or white crystals or as a white crystalline powder. Isoniazid is used in the treatment of tuberculosis. It may be administered orally or intramuscularly. The trade names are Cotinazin, Dinacrin, and Nydrazid.

isoprinosine   An immunomodulator that enhances certain cell-mediated immune functions. It has been shown to have anti-HIV activity in vitro. The drug is available without prescription in several countries, including Mexico. Although it has been popular for self-treatment, isoprinosine's antiviral effects have not consistently correlated with clinical improvement.

Isospora belli infection   Invasion of the body by a species of coccidian protozoa that parasitize the small intestine. Infection is known as coccidiosis. It is generally asymptomatic. When symptoms appear, they may manifest in severe, watery, mucous diarrhea. *See also* coccidiosis.

itch   1) Irritation of the skin, inducing the desire to scratch. 2) Any of a variety of skin disorders characterized by itching. 3) Scabies.

ITP   *see* immune thrombocytopenic purpura

IV   *see* intravenous

IVDA   *see* intravenous drug user

IVDU   *see* intravenous drug user

J

Jaffe, Harold William Born 1946 in Newton, Mass., Jaffe received his M.D. from the University of California, Los Angeles, in 1971. He was part of the original Centers for Disease Control and Prevention task force investigating the outbreak of Pneumocystis carinii pneumonia in homosexual men at the outset of the epidemic. Centers for Disease Control and Prevention, 1600 Clifton Road, N.E., Atlanta, GA 30333, (404) 639-2008.

jaundice A condition characterized by the yellow appearance of the skin, mucous membranes, whites of the eyes, and body fluids and caused by the deposition of bile pigment resulting from too much bilirubin in the blood. *Also called* icterus.

john 1) Slang term for the customer of a prostitute. 2) Slang for any easy mark.

K

Kaposi's sarcoma (KS) 1) A disease affecting especially the skin and mucous membranes that can occur in people with AIDS and others. It is often characterized by the presence of reddish or purplish lesions on the skin. 2) Neoplasms that generally manifest with lymph node involvement or mucocutaneous lesions, particularly in the oral cavity or on the face. Lesions are usually red or purple, may assume varied shapes (round or elliptical), and do not pale under pressure. Internal lesions, especially in the gastrointestinal tract, occur in approximately half of those infected but are most often clinically silent. Neoplasms are generally painless at the onset but may become painful as lesions become more extensive. Therapy is controversial.

Kaposi's Sarcoma Research and Education Foundation *see* San Francisco AIDS Foundation

Kefauver amendments Named after Senator Estes Kefauver, these amendments were passed in 1962 to force the Food and Drug Administration to ensure that drugs were both effective and safe.

ketoconazole A broad-spectrum antifungal agent administered orally and used in the treatment of a variety of fungal infections affecting the skin.

Koop, Charles Everett Born 1916 in Brooklyn, N.Y., Koop received his M.D. from Cornell University in 1941 and his Sc.D. in medicine from the University of Pennsylvania in 1947. A Professor of Pediatric Surgery at the University of Pennsylvania since 1959 and a Professor of Pediatrics since 1976, Koop was Surgeon General for the United States Public Health Service from 1981 to 1989. Children's Hospital, One Children's Center, Philadelphia, PA 19104.

Kramer, Larry   Author, playwright, one of the founders of the Gay Men's Health Crisis and the AIDS Coalition to Unleash Power, and a prominent AIDS activist.

Krim, Mathilde   Born 1926 in Como, Italy, Krim received her Ph.D. in cytogenetics from Geneva University in 1953. Since 1975, an Associate and Member at the Memorial Sloan-Kettering Institute for Cancer Research. She has worked with the American Foundation for AIDS Research since 1988. American Foundation for AIDS Research, 1515 Broadway, Suite 3601, New York, NY 10036.

KS   *see* Kaposi's sarcoma

Kuru disease   A rare disease of the central nervous system isolated in natives of the eastern New Guinea highlands. It is characterized at the onset by a disturbance in muscle coordination, which progresses to paralysis, dementia, and eventual death.

L

Lactobacillus casei factor   *see* folic acid

Lambda Legal Defense and Education Fund   Founded in 1973
to protect the rights of homosexuals in such areas as the administration of justice, child custody, education, employment, housing, and
issues related to AIDS. It seeks to achieve its goals by engaging in test
case litigation, presenting statistics and theoretical information to
courts, educating the legal community about the needs of homosexuals, educating the gay community about legal rights, and providing
assistance to attorneys. The fund maintains a national network of
participating attorneys, operates a speakers' bureau, and sponsors
various seminars. Lambda Legal Defense and Education Fund, 666
Broadway, New York, NY 10012, (212) 995-8585.

Lamblia intestinalis   *see* Giardia lamblia

lambliasis   *see* giardiasis

Langerhans' cell   A star-shaped dendritic cell found primarily in
the epidermis. These cells are believed to be antigen-presenting,
thus participating in certain immune responses.

LAS   *see* lymphadenopathy syndrome

Lasagna, Louis   Born 1923 in New York City, Lasagna received his
M.D. from Columbia University in 1947. He has been the Dean of the
Sackler School of Graduate Biomedical Sciences and Academic Dean
of the Medical School, Tufts University, since 1985. Lasagna chaired
the National Committee to Review Current Procedures for Approval
of New Drugs for Cancer and AIDS. Sackler School of Graduate
Biomedical Sciences, Tufts University, Boston, MA 02111.

Lasagna Committee hearings   *see* National Committee to Review Current Procedures for Approval of New Drugs for Cancer and AIDS

laser therapy   Treatment in surgical procedures using a device that converts various frequencies of light into a single, small, intense, unified beam of monochromatic radiation.

Lassa fever   A disease caused by arenavirus. A native African rat species is a common carrier. Symptoms include acute high fever, abdominal and chest pain, headache, dizziness, cough, nausea, diarrhea, and vomiting. The skin and mucous membranes may begin to hemorrhage. Lassa fever has a relatively high mortality rate in Africa.

latex agglutination test   A test using latex particles as passive carriers of absorbed antigens. The particles clump together after a specific antibody is added.

LAV   *see* lymphadenopathy associated virus

Legionella pneumophila   A species of gram-negative bacteria that causes Legionnaires' disease and Pontiac fever. It has been isolated from numerous locations including tap water, soil, cooling-tower water, aerosolized droplets from heat-exchange systems, human lung tissue, respiratory secretions, and blood.

lentivirus   Any of a group of retroviruses, including those that cause certain diseases in sheep, that affect the pulmonary and central nervous systems.

leprosy   A chronic infectious disease caused by Mycobacterium leprae. It progresses slowly and may manifest itself in various clinical forms. The two principal, or polar, forms are lepromatous and tuberculoid. The lepromatous form is characterized by the development of lesions in the skin and symmetrical involvement of the peripheral nerves, yielding skin anesthesia, muscle weakness, and paralysis. The lepromatous form tends to involve the skin, respiratory tract, and testes. In the tuberculoid form, skin anesthesia occurs early and the nerve lesions are asymmetrical. This form is usually benign. Lepromatous leprosy is much more contagious and malignant than tuberculoid leprosy. Between these two polar forms are the borderline and indeterminant types of leprosy. The borderline form possesses clinical and bacteriological features representing a combination of the two polar forms. The indeterminant group present fewer skin lesions and less abundant bacteria in the lesions.

lesbian   1) An individual who practices lesbianism. 2) A woman whose sexual orientation is toward other women. *Also called* dyke (slang). *See also* homosexual.

lesbianism   Homosexual practice between women. Lesbianism was named after the Island of Lesbos, where sex between women is reported to have been common. *Also called* sapphism after Sappho, a Greek lyric poet of the early 6th century B.C. who lived on the Island of Lesbos.

lesion   1) Any pathologically altered circumscribed area of tissue. 2) An infected area of skin.

leucovorin   *see* folinic acid

leukemia   A chronic or acute disease of the blood-forming elements characterized by the unrestrained growth of leukocytes and their precursors in the blood and bone marrow. Leukemia is classified on the basis of the dominant cell type involved.

leukocyte   A white blood cell or corpuscle. Leukocytes may be classified into two main groups: granulocytes and agranulocytes (nongranular). Granulocytes possess granules in their cytoplasm and include neutrophils, eosinophils, and basophils. Agranulocytes do not possess granules in their cytoplasm and include monocytes and lymphocytes.

leukoencephalopathy   Any of a group of diseases affecting the white matter of the brain.

leukopenia   An abnormal reduction of white blood corpuscles (leukocytes), usually below 5000 per cubic millimeter. Leukopenia may be caused by various infections, drugs, or bone marrow failure.

life cycle   The series of changes in form undergone by any developing organism from its earliest stage to the recurrence of that same stage in the subsequent generation.

Listeria monocytogenes   A species of gram-positive bacteria. In humans, it produces such disorders as meningitis and perinatal septicemia. *Also called* Corynebacterium infantisepticum and Corynebacterium parvulum.

liver Lactobacillus casei factor   *see* folic acid

living will   A document detailing a person's wishes regarding artificial life support in the event of impending death. Living wills are not legal in all states. *See also* durable power of attorney, medical directive, and no code blue.

Lotrimin   *see* clotrimazole

lumbosacral polyradiculopathy   Any of a group of diseases affecting the nerve roots in the lumbar vertebrae and the sacrum (low back region).

lupus anticoagulant   An acquired coagulation inhibitor first noted in patients with systemic lupus erythematosus, but since found in association with other immune disorders, neoplastic disorders, myeloproliferative disorders, pregnancy, and secondary to the administration of certain drugs.

lymphadenopathy   Any disease process in which the lymph nodes are affected and abnormally enlarged.

lymphadenopathy associated virus (LAV)   *see* human immunodeficiency virus

lymphadenopathy syndrome (LAS)   A condition characterized by the presence of unexplained lymphadenopathy for three months or longer. Biopsy reveals nonspecific lymphoid hyperplasia. It is considered by some to be a prodrome (a warning symptom) for the acquired immunodeficiency syndrome.

lymphoblast   A cell that gives rise to a lymphocyte.

lymphocyte   1) A certain type of white blood cell that is essential to the functioning of the immune system. 2) Any of the mononuclear, nonphagocytic leukocytes that make up the body's immunologically competent cells. Found in the blood, lymph, and lymphoid tissues, they are divided on the basis of function and ontogeny. The two main classes are B lymphocytes and T lymphocytes. B lymphocytes are responsible for humoral immunity, and T lymphocytes for cellular immunity. Most are small, with an average of 10 to 12 micrometers in diameter.

lymphocytic interstitial pneumonitis   Inflammation within the lungs that develops gradually and is characterized by infiltration of the lungs by lymphocytes, lymphoblasts, and plasma cells. The cause is unknown, but it is often associated with a compromised immune system. *Also called* lymphoid interstitial pneumonia.

lymphoid interstitial pneumonia   *see* lymphocytic interstitial pneumonitis

lymphokine   A general term used to denote substances released by sensitized lymphocytes on contact with an antigen that are soluble mediators of immune response. They stimulate macrophages and moncytes, assisting with cellular immunity.

lymphoma   A general term used to denote any neoplastic disorder in the lymphatic system. Diseases included under this general group are Hodgkin's disease, lymphatic leukemia, and reticuloses. The term lymphoma is frequently used to denote malignant lymphoma.

lymphoproliferative disease   *see* lymphoproliferative disorder

lymphoproliferative disorder   Any of a group of malignant neoplasms that involve lymphoreticular cells. Included are such disorders as Hodgkin's disease, lymphocytic lymphomas, multiple myeloma, and the histiocytic, lymphocytic, and monocytic leukemias. *Also called* lymphoproliferative disease and lymphoproliferative syndrome.

lymphoproliferative syndrome   *see* lymphoproliferative disorder

lymphoreticular cell   Any reticuloendothelial cell of the lymph node.

lymphotrophic   Having an affinity for lymphatic tissue.

M

macrobiotic diet   A special selection of food and drink designed with the intention of prolonging life.

macrophage   Any of the various forms of mononuclear phagocytes found in loose connective tissues and many organs of the body. Functions of macrophages include nonspecific phagocytosis and pinocytosis, specific pinocytosis of microorganisms that facilitate phagocytosis, killing of ingested microorganisms, digestion and distribution of antigens to B and T lymphocytes, and secretion of various products (e.g., enzymes, prostaglandins, interferon, interleukin-1, complement components, and coagulation factors).

magnetic resonance imaging (MRI)   A technique for providing images of the soft tissues of the body (e.g., heart, brain, large blood vessels) by applying a strong, external, magnetic field that allows for distinguishing between hydrogen atoms in different environments. *Also called* nuclear magnetic resonance imaging (NMRI).

MAI   *see* Mycobacterium avium-intracellular

malignancy   1) A tumor or neoplasm that is not benign. 2) Exhibition (as by a tumor) of a tendency to progress in virulence. 3) The state of being malignant.

malignant   1) Becoming progressively worse; resisting treatment. 2) Tending to produce death; harmful.

malnutrition   1) Any disorder of nutrition. 2) The deficit of efficient or substantive food substances in the body, or the inability to properly absorb food substances and distribute them throughout the body.

mange   1) A skin disease in mammals characterized by itching, lesions, scabs, and loss of hair caused by parasitic mites. 2) A cutaneous communicable disease occurring in various animals including dogs, cats, cattle, horses, sheep, rabbits, rats, and some birds. The causative agent is any of several of the mange mites including Chorioptes, Demodex, Psoroptes, and Sarcoptes. In humans, this condition is known as scabies.

mange mite   Any of the various mites that cause mange.

MAP   *see* Mothers of AIDS Patients

masochism   1) The deriving of sexual pleasure from being dominated, mistreated, or physically abused by one's partner. 2) The deriving of pleasure from suffering physical or psychological pain. *See also* sadism.

mastitis   Inflammation or infection of the breast or mammary gland.

mastoiditis   Inflammation or infection of the air cells of the nipple-shaped portion of the temporal bone (mastoid process).

masturbation   Self-stimulation of the genitals, or other erogenous zones, for sexual pleasure. The term usually applies to self-stimulation to the point of orgasm.

mechanical ventilation   The process of exchanging air between the lungs and surrounding atmosphere by artificial, extrinsic means (i.e., via a respirator).

Medicaid   The U.S. government program designed to provide medical services to the needy and medically needy. It operates through grants to states and is overseen by the Health Care Financing Administration. Administrator, Health Care Financing Administration, Department of Health and Human Services, 200 Independence Avenue, S.W., Washington, DC 20201, (301) 966-3000.

medical directive   A document detailing a patient's wishes concerning kinds of treatment she/he does not wish to have administered. *See also* code blue status, durable power of attorney, living will, no code.

Medicare   The Federal health insurance program, administered by the Health Care Financing Administration, designed to provide medical and hospital care to the elderly (persons over 65) and certain disabled persons such as those in end-stage renal disease. It is funded through social security contributions, premiums, and general revenue. Administrator, Health Care Financing Administration, Department of Health and Human Services, 200 Independence Avenue, S.W., Washington, DC 20201, (301) 966-3000.

megaloblast   A large, abnormal, red blood corpuscle, oval and slightly irregular in shape, from 11 to 20 microns in diameter. They are classified as basophilic, orthochromatic, and polychromatic.

megaloblastic anemia   Anemia characterized by the presence of megaloblasts in the blood and bone marrow.

meninges   The three membranes that ensheathe the brain and spinal cord: the pia mater (internal), the arachnoid (middle), and the dura mater (external).

meningitis   Inflammation or infection of the membranes of the spinal cord and brain (meninges).

meningoencephalitis   Inflammation or infection of the brain and its meninges.

menses   The regular flow of bloody fluid from the genital tract of women. *See also* menstruation.

menstruation   The cyclic discharge of blood and mucosal tissues from the nonpregnant uterus through the vagina. It is brought on by the reduction in production of ovarian hormones and usually recurs in approximately four-week intervals (pending the lack of pregnancy) in the female during the reproductive period (puberty to menopause). It is the culmination of the menstrual cycle.

metabolic acidosis   A disturbance that results in excessive acid in the body fluids due to an increase in acids other than carbonic acid. It may be caused by such conditions as severe infection, dehydration, shock, diarrhea, renal dysfunction, or hepatic dysfunction.

metabolic encephalopathy   Neuropsychiatric disturbances caused by metabolic brain disease. It may be the result of disease in other organs such as the lungs or kidneys, or it may be caused directly by low blood sugar (hypoglycemia), low oxygenation (hypoxia), or decreased blood flow (ischemia).

metastasis   1) Transfer of a disease or its manifestations from one organ or part to another not directly connected with it. 2) Change in location of bacteria or body cells from one part of the body to another.

metastasize   1) To spread to other parts of the body by metastasis. 2) To form new foci of disease in a distant part of the body by metastasis.

methadone   An agent used to detoxify drug addicts. It is a common treatment for heroin addiction.

Meticorten   *see* prednisone

metronidazole   An antiamebic, antibacterial, and antitrichomonal drug appearing as whitish to pale yellowish crystals or crystalline powder. It may be administered orally or intravaginally. The trade name is Flagyl.

Microsporida   An order of parasitic protozoa. *Also called* Cnidosporidia and Microsporidia.

Microsporidia   *see* Microsporida

migrating cheilosis   *see* perleche

milzbrand   *see* anthrax

mineralocorticoid   Any of the biologically active corticosteroids predominantly involved in the regulation of electrolytes and fluid through their effect on ion transport by the renal tubules.

mite   1) Any of a group of small arachnids that are often parasitic. 2) Any arthropod of the order Acarina except the ticks. They are minute arachnids related to the spiders. Some are parasitic and are the causative agent of such conditions as mange or scabies. Others serve as intermediate hosts and carry causative organisms of disease from infected to noninfected individuals.

mitogen   A substance that induces cell division of somatic cells (the cells that become differentiated into the tissues, organs, etc., of the body) in which each daughter cell contains the same number of chromosomes as the parent cell.

molluscum contagiosum   1) A viral infection of the skin. 2) A common, mildly contagious, usually self-limited viral infection of the skin characterized by tumor formations on the skin, affecting mainly children and young adults. The infection is transmitted by autoinoculation, close contact, and any substance that adheres to and transmits infectious materials. It may also affect adults and is usually sexually transmitted in this population. The characteristic lesion is a flesh-colored or gray, navel-shaped papule that progresses to pearly white. The core of the papule contains genetic materials surrounded by a protective coat that serves as a vehicle for replication, and may be expelled.

Moniliaceae   A family of colorless to light-colored, imperfect fungi belonging to the Moniliases order. These include Aspergillus, Blastomyces, Coccidioides, Histoplasma, Penicillum, Sporothrix, Trichoderma, Trichophyton, Trichothecium, and Verticillium.

moniliasis   *see* candidiasis

monoclonal antibody   1) An antibody produced for a specific antigen by a hybridoma. 2) Chemically and immunologically homogenous antibodies derived from hybridoma cells. Their exceptional purity and specificity make them useful as laboratory reagents in various tests (e.g., the ELISA test). They are also used experimentally in cancer immunotherapy.

monocyte   1) A large, mononuclear, nongranular white blood cell. 2) A large, mononuclear, phagocytic leukocyte, with an egg- or kidney-shaped nucleus. They are formed in the bone marrow and transported to tissues (such as those of the liver or lungs), where they develop into macrophages.

mononucleosis   The presence of an abnormally large quantity of mononuclear leukocytes (monocytes) in the blood. The term is often used to refer to infectious mononucleosis.

Montagnier, Luc   Director of the oncogenic viruses unit at the Pasteur Institute. Montagnier and his associates are credited with the discovery of the human immunodeficiency virus. Unite d'Oncologie Virale et U.R.A. 1157, Institut Pasteur, Paris, France.

Mothers of AIDS Patients (MAP)   Founded in 1985, this organization is divided into local groups that provide support for families of persons with AIDS during the illness and after death. It assists with the formation of local groups, functions as a resource network, and conducts educational presentations. Mothers of AIDS Patients, P.O. Box 3132, San Diego, CA 92103, (619) 544-0430.

motor dysfunction   Abnormal, disturbed, or impaired functioning of a muscle, nerve, or center that effects or produces movement.

Motrin   *see* ibuprofen

MRI   *see* magnetic resonance imaging

mucocutaneous infection   The invasion by and multiplication of a pathogenic agent in a mucous membrane or the skin.

mucous membrane   The membrane lining various tubular structures of the body. It consists of a surface layer of epithelium, a basement membrane, and an underlying layer of connective tissue.

multifocal giant-cell encephalitis   *see* AIDS dementia complex

mutation   1) A change or transformation. 2) A permanent variation in genetic structure. 3) A change in the genetic material of a gene that is transmissible to offspring.

myalgia   Tenderness or pain in a muscle or muscles.

Mycelex G   *see* clotrimazole

mycobacterial infection   Invasion by and multiplication of Mycobacteria, the genus that includes the pathogenic causative organisms of tuberculosis and leprosy. These acid-fast organisms are slender, nonmotile, gram-positive rods that do not produce spores or capsules.

Mycobacterium avium-intracellular (MAI)   A complex of slow-growing, nonphotochromogenic organisms that are associated with serious systemic disease in AIDS patients, lymphadenitis in children, human pulmonary disease, and cause tuberculosis in birds and swine.

Mycobacterium kansasii A slow-growing, photochromogenic organism that causes a tuberculosis-like disease in humans.

Mycobacterium leprae The causative agent of leprosy in humans. They typically occur in rounded masses, groups of bacilli, or intracellular clumps.

Mycobacterium tuberculosis A slow-growing, nonphotochromogenic, pathogenic organism that causes tuberculosis in humans, primates, hamsters, guinea pigs, and dogs.

Mycostatin *see* nystatin

myelin 1) A fatlike substance composed of lipids and proteins that coils to form a sheath around the axons of certain nerves and serves as an electrical insulator. 2) A complex lipoid substance found in small quantities in the brain.

myelitis 1) Inflammation of the bone marrow. 2) Inflammation of the spinal cord.

myelopathy 1) A general term denoting any pathological condition of the spinal cord. The term is used to refer to nonspecific lesions, as opposed to inflammatory lesions, which are termed myelitis. 2) Any pathological condition of the bone marrow.

myocardial dysfunction Abnormal, disturbed, or impaired functioning of the muscular tissue of the heart.

myocarditis 1) Inflammation of the middle layer of the heart wall. 2) Inflammation of the muscular walls of the heart.

myositis Inflammation of a muscle, especially a voluntary muscle.

N

NAC   *see* National AIDS Clearinghouse

NAIC   *see* National AIDS Clearinghouse

NAMES Project Foundation   Founded in 1987, this organization was formed to create a patchwork quilt as a memorial to the people who have died as a result of AIDS. The Foundation seeks to emphasize the humanity lost to the pandemic and serves to provide a creative means of expression for those who have been touched by the acquired immunodeficiency syndrome. It produces various publications, raises funds for the care of persons with AIDS, and encourages support for infected individuals and their loved ones. NAMES Project Foundation, P.O. Box 14573, San Francisco, CA 94114, (415) 863-5511.

NAN   *see* National AIDS Network

Naprosyn   *see* naproxen

naproxen   A nonsteroidal, anti-inflammatory drug used for the treatment of osteoarthritis and rheumatoid arthritis. The trade name is Naprosyn.

NAPWA   *see* National Association Of People With AIDS

nasal ulcer   An open sore or lesion of the nose, accompanied by sloughing of inflamed necrotic tissue.

nasopharynx   The part of the pharynx above the soft palate (postnasal area).

National Academy of Sciences   Founded in 1863, an honorary organization that supports the promotion of science and engineering. Members are elected by the Academy in recognition of their contributions to either field. It was founded by an act of Congress to function as the official advisory group on scientific and technical matters and administers the National Academy of Engineering, National Research Council, and Institute of Medicine. National Academy of Sciences, Office of News and Public Information, 2101 Constitution Avenue NW, Washington, DC 20418, (202) 334-2138.

National AIDS Clearinghouse (NAC)   Created for the purpose of disseminating information about the acquired immunodeficiency syndrome, the Clearinghouse distributes free educational materials, maintains a database for service providers, provides information about clinical trials, answers basic reference questions, and houses a resource center for visitors. Formerly called National AIDS Information Clearinghouse. National AIDS Clearinghouse, P.O. Box 6003, 1600 Research Boulevard, Rockville, MD 20850, (800) 458-5231.

National AIDS Information Clearinghouse (NAIC)   *see* National AIDS Clearinghouse

National AIDS Network (NAN)   Founded in 1986, this now defunct organization was formed to link community-based organizations providing education or direct services to those affected by the acquired immunodeficiency syndrome.

National AIDS Research Foundation   An organization set up by Michael Gottlieb in Los Angeles to support AIDS research and to disseminate information about the epidemic. It merged with the AIDS Medical Foundation to form the American Foundation for AIDS Research in 1985.

National Association Of People With AIDS (NAPWA)   Founded in 1985, an organization consisting of individuals who have tested positive to antibodies indicative of infection with the human immunodeficiency virus, who have been diagnosed with AIDS-related complex, or who have been diagnosed with AIDS. The Association works to create, implement, and maintain programs throughout the country designed for self-empowerment, to promote provision of AIDS-related health care, and to expand public understanding of the epidemic. It maintains a speakers' bureau and provides scholarship and grant funding. NAPWA, 2025 I Street, N.W., Suite 415, Washington, DC 20006, (202) 429-2856.

National Cancer Institute (NCI)   A major component of the National Institutes of Health, NCI is the federal government organization responsible for conducting and supporting cancer research. The Institute developed a National Cancer Program to expand existing scientific knowledge on cancer cause and prevention as well as on the diagnosis, treatment, and rehabilitation of cancer patients. Research activities are carried out in-house or are conducted elsewhere and supported through grants or contracts. Cancer research facilities are constructed with Institute support, and training is provided under university-based programs. National Cancer Institute, NIH Building 31, 9000 Rockville Pike, Bethesda, MD 20205, (301) 496-5615.

National Center for Health Statistics (NCHS)   Established in 1960 as a division of the Department of Health and Human Services, the Center collects, analyzes, and disseminates national health statistics; administers the Cooperative Health Statistics System; conducts research; organizes and coordinates the efforts of the various Department of Health and Human Services agencies in health statistics to promote maximum efficiency; cooperates at an international level with organizations concerned with health statistics; functions as a national resource for health data; produces various publications; and sponsors conferences on health statistics. National Center for Health Statistics, Department of Health and Human Services, Public Health Service, Assistant Secretary for Health, 3700 East-West Highway, Hyattsville, MD 20782, (301) 436-7016.

National Commission on AIDS   Created as part of the federal Health Omnibus Programs Extension Act of 1988, the Commission succeeded the Presidential Commission on the Human Immunodeficiency Virus Epidemic. Its purpose is to make recommendations concerning the AIDS epidemic, especially in the area of antidiscrimination legislation. *Also called* Presidential Commission on AIDS.

National Committee to Review Current Procedures for Approval of New Drugs for Cancer and AIDS   Chaired by Dr. Louis Lasagna, the Committee opened in 1989 to review approval procedures for new drugs to be used in the treatment of AIDS and cancer. The parallel track program is an outgrowth of the hearings. *Also called* Lasagna Committee hearings.

National Education Association (NEA)   Founded in 1857, it is a professional organization and union of elementary and secondary school teachers, college and university faculty, administrators, counselors, principals, and other concerned individuals. The Association also produces various publications and sponsors numerous AIDS-prevention programs in schools. National Education Association, 1201 16th Street, N.W., Washington, DC 20036, (202) 833-4000.

National Gay and Lesbian Task Force (NGLTF)   Founded in 1973, this organization is made up of men and women in the United States who are committed to the elimination of prejudice based on sexual orientation. The Task Force offers assistance to individuals and groups working with the homosexual community, produces several publications, and lobbies for gay rights. Formerly called the National Gay Task Force (NGTF). NGLTF, 1517 U Street, N.W., Washington, DC 20009, (202) 332-6483.

National Gay Rights Advocates (NGRA)   Founded in 1978, this public interest law firm was established to promote legal equality for homosexuals. It seeks to achieve this goal by bringing cases to court in order to ensure gay and lesbian civil rights in such areas as employment, immigration, and privacy, and it works to establish legal precedents concerning gay rights. Legal work is free to clients, since law firms and attorneys volunteer their services. It operates the AIDS Civil Rights Project, which has successfully overturned judicial decisions negatively affecting people with AIDS. NGRA produces various publications and provides legal kits for educational purposes, especially in the areas of couples' rights, trusts, and wills. National Gay Rights Advocates, 540 Castro Street, San Francisco, CA 94114, (415) 863-3624.

National Gay Task Force (NGTF)   *see* National Gay and Lesbian Task Force

National Hemophilia Foundation   Founded in 1948, this voluntary organization consists of hemophiliacs, their families, health care professionals, and other concerned individuals. The Foundation sponsors a postgraduate fellowship program to support research, produces various publications, and disseminates information to the public and health care personnel. National Hemophilia Association, 110 Green Street, Room 406, New York, NY 10012, (212) 219-8180.

National Hospice Organization   Founded in 1978, this organization comprises hospice organizations and individuals concerned with the promotion of the hospice concept of care. The organization works to establish standards of care in the planning and implementation of programs, monitors legislation and regulatory acts concerning hospice care, collects data, conducts educational seminars, sponsors professional and peer group networking, and maintains a nonlending library. National Hospice Organization, 1901 N. Moore Street, Suite 901, Arlington, VA 22209, (703) 243-5900.

National Institute of Allergy and Infectious Diseases (NIAID)   Founded in 1948 as a major component of the National Institutes of Health, NIAID conducts and supports broadly based research and research training in the causes, characteristics, prevention, control, and treatment of a wide variety of diseases believed to be attributable to infectious agents (including bacteria, viruses, and parasites), allergies, or other deficiencies and disorders in the responses of the body's immune mechanisms. NIAID, NIH Building 31, 9000 Rockville Pike, Bethesda, MD 20205, (301) 496-5717.

National Institute of Justice (NIJ)   Founded in 1968, the Institute is the primary federal sponsor of research on crime and its control and is a central resource for information on innovative approaches to criminal justice. It sponsors and conducts research, evaluates policies and practices, demonstrates promising new approaches, provides training and technical assistance, assesses new technology for criminal justice, and disseminates its findings at the state and local levels. National Institute of Justice, Department of Justice, 633 Indiana Avenue, N.W., Washington, DC 20531, (202) 724-2942.

National Institute of Mental Health (NIMH)   Founded in 1948, the Institute provides a national focus for the federal effort to increase knowledge and advance effective strategies to deal with health problems and issues in the promotion of mental health and prevention and treatment of mental illness. It conducts and supports research; provides technical assistance to various organizations; collects, analyzes, and disseminates data; and carries out administrative and financial management functions necessary to implement programs. National Institute of Mental Health, Department of Health and Human Services, Public Health Service, Alcohol, Drug, and Mental Health Administration, 5600 Fishers Lane, Rockville, MD 20857, (301) 443-3673.

National Institute on Drug Abuse (NIDA)   Founded in 1972, the Institute provides a national focus for the federal effort to increase knowledge and promote effective strategies in dealing with health problems and issues associated with drug abuse. NIDA conducts and supports research; supports research training and career development; provides technical assistance at various levels; collaborates with organizations and institutions to facilitate and extend programs for the prevention of drug abuse and addiction and for the care, treatment, and rehabilitation of drug abusers; and carries out administrative and financial management functions necessary for the implementation of programs. National Institute on Drug Abuse, Department of Health and Human Services, Public Health Service Alcohol, Drug Abuse, and Mental Health Administration, 5000 Fishers Lane, Rockville, MD 20857, (301) 443-6480.

National Institutes of Health (NIH)   NIH is the primary medical research branch of the federal government, with a mission to improve the health of the American people. To carry out this mission, the agency conducts and supports biomedical research into the causes, prevention, and cure of diseases; supports research training and the development of research resources; and makes use of modern methods to communicate biomedical information. It is organized into the Fogarty International Center, the Clinical Center, the National Library of Medicine, four divisions (Computer Research and Technology, Research Grants, Research Resources, and Research Services), and twelve research institutions (National Cancer Institute; National Heart, Lung, and Blood Institute; National Institute of Arthritis; National Institute of Diabetes, and Digestive and Kidney Diseases; National Institute of Allergy and Infectious Diseases; National Institute of Child Health and Human Development; National Institute of Dental Research; National Institute of Environmental Health Sciences; National Institute of General Medical Sciences; National Institute of Neurological and Communicative Disorders and Stroke; National Eye Institute; and National Institute on Aging). National Institutes of Health, Department of Health and Human Services, Public Health Service, 9000 Rockville Pike, Bethesda, MD 20892.

National Leadership Coalition on AIDS   Founded in 1987, this organization functions as a clearinghouse on the issue of AIDS in the workplace. It serves the business and labor communities, while attempting to increase involvement by these groups in the fight against the spread of HIV. The Coalition produces several publications and maintains an on-site library. National Leadership Coalition on AIDS, 1150 17th Street, N.W., Suite 202, Washington, DC 20036, (202) 429-0930.

National Lesbian and Gay Health Foundation (NLGHF)   Founded in 1980, this organization comprises health care professionals providing services to homosexuals and individuals concerned with the quality and availability of care for lesbians and gays. The Foundation seeks to create, establish, and coordinate interdisciplinary programs and activities to promote a healthier environment for the homosexual community and to expand the delivery of appropriate care. It promotes and supports research, serves as a liaison at various levels, provides educational services, conducts training programs, compiles statistics, maintains a speakers' bureau, disseminates AIDS information, and sponsors the National Association of People With AIDS. NLGHF, P.O. Box 65472, Washington, DC 20035, (202) 797-3708.

National Library of Medicine (NLM)   The Library, which serves as the nation's chief medical information source, is authorized to provide medical library services and online bibliographic searching capabilities, such as MEDLINE, AIDSLINE, AIDSTRIALS, AIDS-DRUGS, and others, to public and private agencies and organizations, institutions, and individuals. It is responsible for the development and management of a Biomedical Communications Network, applying advanced technology to the improvement of biomedical communications, and operates a computer-based toxicology information system for the scientific community, industry, and other federal agencies. Through grants and contracts, the Library administers programs of assistance to the nation's medical libraries that include support of a Regional Medical Library network, research in the field of medical library science, establishment and improvement of basic library resources, and supporting nonprofit biomedical scientific publications. National Library of Medicine, National Institutes of Health, Department of Health and Human Services, Public Health Service, 8600 Rockville Pike, Bethesda, MD 20209, (301) 496-6308.

National Minority AIDS Council (NMAC)   Founded in 1986, this organization is divided into local, state, and regional groups that seek to address AIDS issues as they affect minority communities and to support and promote education for minorities. It maintains a speakers' bureau, on-site library, and biographical archives; compiles statistics; produces various publications; and conducts educational and training programs. The Council is headquartered at 3001 I Street, N.W., Suite 400, Washington, DC 20002, (202) 544-1076.

National Mobilization Against AIDS   Founded in 1984, this organization seeks to increase government funding of AIDS-related services and promote public support of persons with AIDS. It maintains a speakers' bureau for addressing the impact of the AIDS pandemic on civil rights.

National Resource Center on Women and AIDS   Founded in 1988, this organization functions as a clearinghouse for issues involving women and AIDS. It conducts research, maintains a speakers' bureau, provides educational and technical support, and produces several publications. National Resource Center on Women and AIDS, 2000 P Street, N.W., Suite 508, Washington, DC 20036, (202) 872-1770.

natural killer cells (NK cells)   Large, granular lymphocytes that attach themselves to virus-infected cells. The natural killer cells attack and destroy the virus by secreting cytotoxic molecules. They are also effective against some tumor cells. This process is one of the earliest immune defense mechanisms against viral infections.

NCHS   *see* National Center for Health Statistics

NCI   *see* National Cancer Institute

NDA   *see* New Drug Application

NEA   *see* National Education Association

necropsy   *see* autopsy

necrosis   1) The death of areas of tissue. 2) The constellation of morphological changes indicative of cell death and caused by the progressive degenerative action of various enzymes.

needle sharing   The act, practice, or process of using a hypodermic syringe in common with another person or persons. Generally the term is applied to drug addicts who reuse a needle after someone else, without sterilizing it, for the purpose of injecting intravenous drugs.

needle-exchange program   Any program established for intra-venous drug users educating them or enabling them to exchange used needles and syringes for sterile ones. These programs have been created in an effort to remove contaminated works from this commu-nity and reduce the spread of the human immunodeficiency virus via this route of transmission.

needlestick   The unintentional puncture of the skin with a hypo-dermic needle.

nef gene   The gene in the human immunodeficiency virus that encodes proteins of 27,000 molecular weight and effects virus replica-tion by decreasing virus production.

Neisseria gonorrhoeae   A species of gram-negative bacteria be-longing to the genus Neisseria that cause gonorrhea.

neonate   1) A newborn infant. 2) Newly born.

neoplasm   Any new and abnormal formation of tissue, such as a growth or tumor. The growth is uncontrolled, progressive, and serves no useful function.

neoplastic   Pertaining to, or of the nature of, a neoplasm; pertain-ing to new, abnormal tissue formation.

neurologic complication   A disease or abnormality of the nerv-ous system that is superimposed upon another disease without being specifically related to it, yet affecting or modifying the prognosis of the original disease.

neurologic dysfunction   Abnormal, disturbed, or impaired func-tioning of the nervous system.

neurology   The branch of science dealing with the study of the nervous system and its disorders.

neuropathology   The branch of medicine that deals with the study of diseases of the nervous system, as well as microscopic and macro-scopic structural and functional changes occurring in them.

neuropathy   1) A general term used to denote pathological changes or dysfunction in the peripheral nervous system. 2) A term used to denote any disease of the nerves.

neuropsychiatric complication   A nervous or mental disease or difficulty superimposed upon another disease without being specifically related to it, yet affecting or modifying the prognosis of the original disease.

neuropsychiatry   The branch of medicine concerned with the study of nervous and mental disorders.

neurosyphilis   Syphilis affecting the central nervous system. It may be divided into two groups: asymptomatic and symptomatic.

neutropenia   A decrease in the number of neutrophil cells in the blood.

neutrophil   1) A granular leukocyte (white blood cell or corpuscle) with the properties of adherence to immune complexes, chemotaxis, and phagocytosis. It is readily stainable with neutral dyes. 2) Any cell, structure, or histologic element that stains easily with neutral dye.

New Drug Application (NDA)   The status awarded a drug by the Food and Drug Administration that allows it to be sold for profit.

NGLTF   *see* National Gay and Lesbian Task Force

NGRA   *see* National Gay Rights Advocates

NGTF   *see* National Gay and Lesbian Task Force

NIAID   *see* National Institute of Allergy and Infectious Diseases

NIDA   *see* National Institute on Drug Abuse

night sweat   Profuse sweating at night during sleep. It is sometimes an early sign of disease.

NIH   *see* National Institutes of Health

NIJ   *see* National Institute of Justice

NIMH   *see* National Institute of Mental Health

NK cells   *see* natural killer cells

NLGHF   *see* National Lesbian and Gay Health Foundation

NLM   *see* National Library of Medicine

NMAC   *see* National Minority AIDS Council

NMRI   *see* magnetic resonance imaging

no code   An indication on a terminally ill patient's chart that he/ she does not want heroic, life-saving measures or artificial life support when death is imminent. *Also called* no code blue or no code blue status. *See also* durable power of attorney, medical directive, and living will.

no code blue   *see* no code

no code blue status   *see* no code

Nocardia   A genus of aerobic, nonmotile actinomycetes that are transitional between bacteria and fungi. Most forms exist on dead organic matter, and some may produce disease in humans. *See* nocardiosis.

nocardia   A vernacular term used to denote any member of the genus Nocardia.

nocardiosis   An acute or chronic pathological condition caused by infection from any species of Nocardia. It may occur as a pulmonary infection but has a marked tendency to spread to any organ of the body, especially the brain. It results in abscesses in the lungs, brain, skin, or other areas.

node   1) A knot, knob, protuberance, or swelling. 2) A small mass of tissue in the form of a knot or swelling.

nodular lesion   A circumscribed area of pathologically altered tissue that possesses the characteristics of a nodule.

nodule   A small knot or protuberance that can be detected by touch.

non-Hodgkin's lymphoma   A lymphoma other than Hodgkin's disease. They may be classified into nodular or diffuse tumor patterns and by cell type; or into high-, intermediate-, and low-grade malignancy and into cytologic subtypes.

nonoxynol-9   A spermicide found in many lubricants and in some condoms that has been found to kill the human immunodeficiency virus. It is often recommended (along with condoms) to help reduce the risk of HIV transmission. *See also* safe sex.

Northern blot technique   A procedure to separate and identify RNA fragments. They are separated by electrophoresis on an agarose gel, blotted onto a nitrocellulose or nylon membrane, and hybridized with labeled nucleic acid probes.

Norwegian scabies   A rare, severe form of scabies characterized by an extremely heavy infestation of mites that appears in patients with poor sensation, severe systemic disease, senility or mental retardation, and immunosuppression.

Novello, Antonia Coello   Born in Fajardo, Puerto Rico, in 1944, Novello received her M.D. from the University of Puerto Rico School of Medicine in 1970, her master's degree in public health from Johns Hopkins University in 1982, and her certification from the John F. Kennedy School of Government, Harvard University, in 1987. Since 1986, she has been the Deputy Director, General Pediatrics and Obstetrics and Gynecology, National Institute of Child Health and Human Development, National Institutes of Health. She is the current Surgeon General for the United States Public Health Service. Office address: 1315 31st Street, N.W., Washington, DC 20007.

nuclear magnetic resonance imaging   *see* magnetic resonance imaging

nucleoside   A glycoside (any of a group of sugar derivatives that, when combined with water, yields a sugar and one or more other substances) formed by the combination of a sugar (pentose) and a purine or pyrimide base.

Nuprin   *see* ibuprofen

Nydrazid   *see* isoniazid

nystatin   An antibiotic appearing as a yellowish to tan powder. It is an antifungal used in the treatment of cutaneous, intestinal, oral, or vaginal candidal infections. Nystatin may be administered orally or topically. *Also called* fungicidin. The trade names are Mycostatin and O-V Statin.

O

O-V Statin *see* nystatin

occupational exposure The risk of exposure to a communicable disease through the normal procedures associated with a specific profession (e.g., a needlestick during a surgical procedure).

Occupational Safety and Health Administration (OSHA) Established pursuant to the Occupational Safety and Health Act of 1970, it develops and promulgates occupational safety and health standards, develops and issues regulations, conducts investigations and inspections to determine the status of compliance with regulations, issues citations, and proposes penalties for noncompliance. Occupational Safety and Health Administration, Department of Labor, 200 Constitution Avenue, N.W., Washington, DC 20210, (202) 523-8017.

odynophagia Pain upon swallowing.

Office of Management and Budget (OMB) Established in 1970 as part of the Executive Office of the President pursuant to Recognition Plan No. 2, the OMB evaluates, formulates, and coordinates management procedures and program objectives within and among federal departments and agencies. It also controls the administration of the federal budget, while routinely providing the president with recommendations regarding budget proposals and relevant legislative enactments. Office of Management and Budget, Executive Office Building, Washington, DC 20503, (202) 395-3080.

OI *see* opportunistic infection

oidomycosis *see* candidiasis

OMB   *see* Office of Management and Budget

Omnipen   *see* ampicillin

oncogene   A gene found in the chromosomes of tumor cells that has the ability to induce a normal cell to become malignant.

oncology   The study of tumors.

oocyst   The encysted form of the fertilized macrogamete, or zygote, in coccidian sporozoa in which sporogonic multiplication occurs. This results in the formation of infectious agents (sporozoites) for the next stage of sporozoan life cycle.

opportunistic infection (OI)   Invasion and multiplication of microorganisms (especially fungi and bacteria) that under ordinary circumstances do not cause disease but in certain instances become pathogenic. Individuals with impaired immune responses (such as persons with AIDS) are especially susceptible to opportunistic infections. The infection occurs because the altered physiological state of the host provides the opportunity. In some instances, as when antibiotics are administered over a prolonged period, some microorganisms that ordinarily do not cause disease become pathogenic because of the continued suppression of the more prevalent microorganism.

oral candida   Candidal infection of the mouth. *See also* Candida.

oral candidiasis   Infection of the skin or mucous membranes in the mouth with any species of Candida. *Also called* pseudomembranous candidiasis and thrush. *See also* candidiasis.

oral lesion   A circumscribed area of pathologically altered tissue or skin in the mouth.

oral sex   Sexual activity in which the genitalia are stimulated with the tongue and mouth.

Orasone   *see* prednisone

ornithosis   *see* psittacosis

OSHA   *see* Occupational Safety and Health Administration

otitis media   Inflammation of the middle ear.

otopharyngeal complication   A disease involving the ear and pharynx that is superimposed upon another disease without being specifically related to it, yet affecting or modifying the prognosis of the original disease.

ovine-caprine lentiviruses   Any of the lentiviruses associated with sheep or goats.

P

PAC *see* Pediatric AIDS Coalition

pachydermatosis *see* elephantiasis

paleopathology The study of diseases as found in remains of bodies still extant from ancient times.

pancreatitis Acute or chronic inflammation of the pancreas. It may be symptomatic or asymptomatic and is most often caused by alcoholism, biliary tract disease, or adverse reaction to the administration of a drug.

pandemic 1) Occuring over a wide geographic area and affecting a large number of people. 2) An epidemic occuring over a wide geographic area and affecting a large number of people.

papillary tumor *see* papilloma

papilloma 1) A benign tumor of the skin or mucous membrane. 2) Any benign epithelial neoplasm. Warts are included in this group. *Also called* papillary tumor, villoma, and villous papilloma or villous tumor. *See also* papillomavirus.

papillomavirus Any of a group of viruses that cause papillomas in man and animals. They are a subgroup of the papovaviruses.

papovavirus Any of a group of viruses, many of which are oncogenic (capable of causing a normal cell to become cancerous) that are involved in viral carcinogenesis (cancer production). Included in this group are papillomaviruses and polyomaviruses.

119

papule   A small, circumscribed, elevated, solid, superficial area on the skin.

papulosquamous disease   Any pathological condition of the body characterized by papules and scales, such as psoriasis or seborrheic dermatitis.

parallel track   The provision of an alternative track for the administration of experimental drugs to individuals who do not qualify for clinical trials. This alternative program is an outgrowth of the hearings of the National Committee to Review Current Procedures for Approval of New Drugs for Cancer and AIDS chaired by Dr. Louis Lasagna.

parasite   A plant or animal that lives upon, within, or at the expense of another living organism (host) without contributing to that organism's survival. *See also* host.

parotiditis   *see* parotitis

parotitis   Inflammation of the parotid gland. *Also called* parotiditis.

paroxysmal   1) Occurring in sudden, periodic attacks. 2) Spasmodic, convulsive.

parrot fever   *see* psittacosis

partner notification   The act of informing one's sexual partner(s) as to the status of one's health (e.g., divulging that fact that an individual has tested positive for the presence of the human immunodeficiency virus).

passive anal intercourse   *see* receptive anal intercourse

Pasteur Institute   Founded in 1888, it is considered to be the first institute of large, independent, public hygiene research organizations. When founded, it served definite practical purposes and performed basic research. The Institute currently conducts basic and applied research in biology and medicine including such fields as biochemistry, cellular and molecular biology, developmental biology, immunology, microbiology, mycology, pharmacology, protozoology, and virology. Pasteur Institute, 25-28 rue du Doctor Roux, 75015 Paris, France.

Pasteurella multocida   1) A bacteria common to the mouth and respiratory tract. 2) A small, nonmotile, gram-negative bacteria that is part of the normal flora of the mouth and respiratory tract of animals and birds. Human disease usually results from an animal bite or scratch, with abscesses, bacteremia, bronchiectasis, localized swelling, meningitis, pneumonia, and septicemia being common symptoms.

patent   1) An official document open to public examination and granting a certain right or privilege, especially the right to produce, sell, or gain profit from an invention, process, or product for a specified number of years. 2) To secure the exclusive right to produce, use, or sell by a patent.

pathogen   Any agent, especially a microorganism, capable of causing disease.

pathogenesis   1) The origin and development of a disease. 2) The cellular events and reactions culminating in the development of a disease.

pathogenic   Producing disease.

pathological   1) Of pathology. 2) Due to or involving disease.

pathology   1) The branch of medicine concerned with the nature of disease, especially the functional and structural changes caused by disease. 2) Any conditions, process, or results of a particular disease.

pathophysiology   The study of how normal functions of the living organism and its components are altered by disease.

patient   1) An individual who is ill or undergoing treatment for disease or injury. 2) A person receiving medical care.

patient autonomy   The condition in which the patient maintains control over the direction of her/his treatment.

PCP   *see* Pneumocystis carinii pneumonia

pediatric AIDS   The condition involving the acquired immunodeficiency syndrome in individuals between birth and age 13. *See also* acquired immunodeficiency syndrome.

Pediatric AIDS Coalition (PAC)   This advocacy group seeks to promote AIDS treatment, research, and education for children. It is located at 1331 Pennsylvania Avenue, N.W., Suite 721-N, Washington, DC 20004, (202) 662-7460.

peliosis hepatis   A condition characterized by blue patches on the liver. It is caused by blood-filled spaces in those parts of the liver that are concerned with its function rather than its structure.

pelvic inflammatory disease (PID)   Inflammation in the pelvic cavity. It may be acute or chronic and often involves pus-forming lesions in the female genital tract.

penicillin   A large group of antibacterial antibiotics that are biosynthesized by several species of molds of the genus Penicillium. Produced naturally as well as synthetically, penicillin is especially effective on gram-positive bacteria. It is also active on certain gram-negative pathogens.

Penicillium   A genus of fungi, with certain species yielding antibiotic substances and biologicals (e.g., Penicillium chrysogenum yields penicillin).

pentamidine   A drug used in the treatment of Pneumocystis carinii pneumonia. *See also* aerosolized pentamidine and pentamidine isethionate.

pentamidine isethionate   A toxic drug effective in the treatment of Pneumocystis carinii pneumonia and also used in the prophylaxis and treatment of early stages of African sleeping sickness. Since it does not cross the blood-brain barrier, it is not effective in the advanced stage of this disease.

Pentatrichomonas hominis   A species of parasitic protozoan flagellates belonging to the genus Pentatrichomonas that live as a commensal in the colon of humans and a variety of animals. Formerly called Trichomonas hominis.

pentose   A monosaccharide (a carbohydrate not decomposable by hydrolysis) containing five carbon atoms in the molecule (e.g., arabinose, ribose).

People With AIDS Coalition   Founded in 1985, the Coalition comprises local support networks for people with AIDS. It conducts research, operates a speakers' bureau, maintains a library, produces various publications, serves as a liaison to social service organizations, and operates a drop-in service. People with AIDS Coalition, 31 W. 26th Street, New York, NY 10011, (212) 532-0290.

Peptide T   A small polypeptide (a substance containing two or more amino acids in the molecule joined together by peptide linkages) that has been reported, in the laboratory, to block the binding of HIV to the surface of susceptible cells. Research is in progress to confirm the in vitro studies, and an investigational new drug status has been granted by the Food and Drug Administration allowing for Phase I clinical trails.

percutaneous   Performed through the skin (e.g., injection or removal accomplished by a needle inserted through the skin).

pericarditis   Inflammation of the pericardium (the outside lining of the heart).

pericardium   The fibroserous sac enclosing the heart and the origins of the great blood vessels. It consists of an inner serous layer (epicardium or visceral pericardium) and an outer layer of fibrous tissue (parietal pericardium). The base of the pericardium is attached to the diaphragm.

perinatal   The period shortly before and after birth. Definitions vary widely: from the 28th week of pregnancy through seven days after birth (in its shortest form) to the 20th week of gestation through 28 days after birth (in its longest form).

periodontal disease   Any pathologic condition of the supporting structures of the teeth (periodontium).

peritoneal cavity   A potential space between layers of the parietal and visceral peritoneum.

peritoneal dialysis   Dialysis in which the lining of the peritoneal cavity is used as the dialysis membrane. The dialyzing solution is introduced into and removed from the peritoneal cavity.

peritoneum   The serous membrane reflected over the viscera and lining the abdominopelvic walls.

peritonitis   Inflammation or infection of the peritoneum. It is accompanied by abdominal pain, constipation, vomiting, and fever.

perleche   A disorder marked by single or multiple fissures and cracks at the corners of the mouth. In advanced stages, it may spread to the lips and cheeks. It may be due to oral candidiasis, a dietary deficiency, poor hygiene, drooling of saliva, or other causes. *Also called* angular cheilitis, angular cheilosis, angular stomatitis, migrating cheilosis, and intertrigo labialis.

persistent generalized lymphadenopathy (PGL)   Lymph node enlargement of one centimeter or greater at two or more extrainguinal sites and persisting for more than three months without a concurrent illness, condition, or any explanation other than infection with the human immunodeficiency virus. PGL constitutes Group III of the Centers for Disease Control and Prevention's classification system for HIV infection.

person living with AIDS (PLWA)   *see* person with AIDS

person with AIDS (PWA)   An individual who is infected with the human immunodeficiency virus and has manifested one of the predefined opportunistic infections or diseases that qualify for an AIDS diagnosis. *Also called* person living with AIDS (PLWA). *See also* acquired immunodeficiency syndrome.

person with AIDS-related complex (PWARC)   An individual exhibiting signs and symptoms indicative of the AIDS-related complex (e.g., fever, persistent generalized lymphadenopathy, and weight loss accompanied by HIV infection). *See also* AIDS-related complex and acquired immunodeficiency syndrome.

personal hygiene   1) An individual's practices used for the preservation of health and prevention of disease. 2) Cleanliness, sanitary practices.

PGL   *see* persistent generalized lymphadenopathy

PHA   *see* phytohemagglutinin

phagocyte   Any cell that ingests and destroys other cells, microorganisms, or other foreign matter in the blood or tissues.

phagocytosis   The process of cells engulfing, ingesting, and digesting solid substances such as bacteria, other cells, or foreign particles.

pharmacology   The branch of science dealing with the study of the origin, nature, properties, uses, and effects of drugs.

Phase I   The classification of clinical trials designed to determine the safety of an experimental drug and to gauge the most effective dosage.

Phase II   The classification of clinical trials designed to test the efficacy (effectiveness) of an experimental drug and to examine any side effects caused by that drug. Phase II trials often are conducted using large numbers of participants who are randomly administered either the experimental drug or a placebo. These randomized, controlled trials generally are double-blind (i.e., no one knows which participants are receiving the drug until after the study).

phosphonoformate   An antiviral drug approved by the Food and Drug Administration for the treatment of cytomegalovirus retinitis. The trade name is Foscarnet.

phytohemagglutinin (PHA)   A lectin found in the red kidney bean that agglutinates (joins by adhesion) erythrocytes and stimulates predominantly T lymphocytes.

PI   *see* Project Inform or principal investigator

PID   *see* pelvic inflammatory disease

pinocytosis   The cellular process of actively engulfing liquid.

piritrexim   1) A folic acid antagonist. 2) A lipid-soluble antifolate shown to have activity against both Pneumocystis carinii and Toxoplasma gondii. Studies are currently under way to judge the effectiveness of this drug.

Pitressin   *see* vasopressin

placebo   An inactive substance with no medical value, initially administered for the sole purpose of satisfying a patient's psychophysiological craving for medication. More recently, placebos have been administered to control groups in clinical trials in order to distinguish the effects of experimental treatment. *See also* control group and clinical trial.

plasmacytosis   An excess of plasma cells in the blood.

plasmapheresis   The separation of the cellular elements of the blood from the plasma after it has been withdrawn from the body. The packed red cells are then retransfused into the donor, or to an individual requiring red cells rather than whole blood.

PLWA   *see* person with AIDS

pneumococcal vaccine   A vaccine that induces immunity against certain capsule types of disease caused by the pneumococcus bacterium.

pneumococcus   An oval-shaped, encapsulated, non-spore-forming, gram-positive organism causing such infections as pneumonia, mastoiditis, otitis media, bronchitis, meningitis, keratitis, bloodstream infections, and conjunctivitis.

Pneumocystis carinii   1) The causative agent of Pneumocystis carinii pneumonia. 2) A genus of microorganisms that cause the acute interstitial cell pneumonia, Pneumocystis carinii pneumonia.

Pneumocystis carinii pneumonia (PCP)   Protozoal infection of the pulmonary system which generally presents symptoms of fever, cough, difficulty or pain in breathing, and tightness of the chest. It is the leading cause of death among people with AIDS. Trimethoprim-sulfamethoxazole and pentamidine isethionate are both used as standard drug therapies.

pneumonia   Inflammation of the lungs, caused primarily by bacteria, chemical irritants, and viruses, and resulting in solidification of the lung tissue

pneumonitis   Inflammation of the lungs. *See also* pneumonia.

podophyllotoxin A highly toxic compound that has cathartic and antineoplastic properties.

pol gene The gene that encodes the reverse transcriptase enzyme of the human immunodeficiency virus, transcribes viral RNA into DNA, and encodes a portion of the HIV protease and an endonuclease protein.

poliomyelitis vaccine *see* poliovirus vaccine inactivated

poliovirus vaccine inactivated A suspension of three types of inactivated poliovirus (I, II, III) used both in the immunization of unimmunized adults and for immunologically deficient patients. *Also called* poliomyelitis vaccine and Salk vaccine.

Polycillin *see* ampicillin

Polymox *see* amoxicillin

polyneuropathy A disease that involves a number of nerves.

polyomavirus Any of a subgroup of the papovaviruses that causes malignancies in lower animals (e.g., mice).

Popham, Paul One of the founders and former president of the Gay Men's Health Crisis. Popham died of an AIDS-related illness.

poppers *see* amyl nitrite inhalant and butyl nitrite inhalant

porphyria Any of a group of disturbances in porphyrin metabolism characterized by increased formation and excretion of porphyrins or their precursors.

porphyrin Any of a group of nitrogen-containing organic compounds, obtained from chlorophyll and hemoglobin, that occur in protoplasm and form the basis of respiratory pigments in plants and animals.

postmortem examination *see* autopsy

postpartum Occurring after childbirth or delivery. The term refers to the mother.

postural hypotension   A decrease in blood pressure upon rising to an erect position or posture. Although normal, it may cause fainting under certain conditions (may result from rising after having been bedridden for several days). *See also* blackout.

power of attorney   A written statement legally authorizing a person to act on behalf of another. *See also* durable power of attorney.

prednisone   A steroid hormone derived from cortisone. It is administered orally to treat various conditions that respond to the anti-inflammatory properties of this type of hormone. *Also called* deltacortisone. The trade names are Deltasone, Meticorten, Orasone, and SK-Prednisone.

premarital testing   Testing prior to marriage for the presence of antibodies indicative of specific diseases.

Prencipen   *see* ampicillin

prepartum   Occurring just before childbirth.

Presidential Commission on AIDS   *see* Presidential Commission on the Human Immunodeficiency Virus Epidemic and National Commission on AIDS

Presidential Commission on the Human Immunodeficiency Virus Epidemic   Established by President Reagan in 1987, the Commission was founded to make recommendations at the federal level concerning the HIV epidemic, especially antidiscrimination legislation. It was succeeded in 1988 by the National Commission on AIDS. *Also called* Presidential Commission on AIDS and Watkins Commission.

presumptive diagnosis   1) A diagnosis based on reasonable grounds for conclusions established by previous, commonly accepted experience. This procedure may be used when diagnostic tests are not available or cannot be obtained. 2) The opposite of definitive diagnosis.

prevalence   The number of cases of a disease present in a population at a specific point in time. *See also* incidence.

principal investigator (PI)   The director of a research project that is either partially or fully supported by grant funding.

proctitis   Inflammation of the anus and rectum. Blood, mucus, or pus may be present in the excrement.

proctocolitis   Inflammation of the colon and rectum. *Also called* coloproctitis.

prognosis   1) The forecast or prediction as to the course and outcome of a disease. 2) The estimate of recovery from a disease based on the conditions exhibited by the case.

progressive multifocal leukoencephalopathy   A disease in which destruction of the myelin sheath of the nerve is usually found in the white matter of the brain, but rarely in the brain stem and cerebellum. It occurs secondary to various neoplastic diseases and is generally fatal.

Project Inform (PI)   Founded in 1985, it was established to disseminate information concerning experimental treatments for the acquired immunodeficiency syndrome or the human immunodeficiency virus and to lobby for expanded research and health care services in this area. Project Inform, 347 Dolores Street, Suite 301, San Francisco, CA 94110, (800) 822-7422, (800) 334-7422 (California only).

promiscuity   1) The state, quality, or instance of exercising a lack of discrimination, specifically with reference to engaging in sexual activities. 2) The state, quality, or instance of casually engaging in sexual intercourse with one or more people.

prophylaxis   The prevention of disease; treatment to prevent disease.

prostitute   A man or woman who engages in sexual intercourse for pay. *Also called* hooker (slang).

protocol   A detailed plan of an experiment.

protozoa   The subkingdom that includes the simplest organisms of the animal kingdom. It consists of unicellular organisms that range in size from submicroscopic to macroscopic. Reproduction is usually asexual by fission, but conjugation and sexual reproduction do occur. Most are free-living, but some exist as commensals, mutualists, or parasites.

protozoal infection   The state or condition in which the body is invaded by protozoa.

protozoan   1) Concerning or pertaining to protozoa. 2) An individual of the protozoa.

pruritic papule   A pale, dome-shaped, intensely itchy lesion with a small vesicle on top which progresses to crusting.

pseudomembranous candidiasis   *see* oral candidiasis

psittacosis   An acute or chronic respiratory and systemic infectious disease that is caused by Chlamydia psittaci. Although it affects primarily parrots and other birds, it may be transmitted to humans. Human infection is generally caused by inhaling dried, contaminated bird excreta, or occasionally by handling bird products containing the pathogen. Infection may be asymptomatic. When symptoms appear, they range from a mild influenza-like manifestation to a severe and fatal pneumonia. *Also called* ornithosis and parrot fever.

psoriasis   1) A chronic skin disease characterized by scaly, reddish patches. 2) A common, autoimmune, chronic, inflammatory disease of the skin characterized by flare-ups and remissions and consisting of erythematous papules that come together to form plaques with distinct borders. It has an affinity for the extensor surfaces, genitalia, lumbosacral region, nails, and scalp. If the disease is untreated and progression continues, silvery to yellow-white scales may develop. Severity of the disease ranges from a minimal cosmetic problem to total body involvement and sometimes can be life-threatening (psoriatic erythroderma).

psychosis   A mental disorder characterized by personality disintegration and gross impairment of perception and contact with reality. The disturbances are generally marked by delusions, hallucinations, and incoherent speech. The term may also be applied, in a more general sense, to refer to disorders in which impaired mental functioning results in an interference with the patient's ability to cope with the daily demands of life.

psychosocial issue A result, consequence, or outcome relating to both psychological and social factors.

pteroylglutamic acid *see* folic acid

pulmonary alveolar proteinosis A chronic lung disease of unknown cause in which eosinophilic material is deposited in the alveoli. This prevents ventilation of the affected areas. It is characterized by dyspnea (shortness of breath or difficulty in breathing), chest pain, weakness, and weight loss. Pulmonary insufficiency may lead to death.

pulmonary dysfunction Abnormal, disturbed, or impaired functioning of the lungs.

purine A colorless, crystalline, heterocyclic compound that is the parent compound of purine bases (e.g., adenine, caffeine, guanine, uric acid, and xanthine).

purpura A small hemorrhage (up to one centimeter in diameter) in the skin, mucous membranes, internal organs, and other tissues resulting from varied causes including blood disorders, trauma, and vascular abnormalities.

PWA *see* person with AIDS

PWARC *see* person with AIDS-related complex

pyrimethamine An antiviral drug appearing as a white crystalline powder. It is used in the prophylaxis of malaria and in conjunction with a sulfonamide in the treatment of toxoplasmosis. Pyrimethamine is administered orally. The trade name is Daraprim.

pyrimethamine/sulfadiazine Combined drug therapy using pyrimethamine and sulfadiazine.

Q

quarantine   1) Any isolation or restriction of movement imposed on people to prevent or control the spread of an infectious disease. 2) The period of detention of a ship upon entering a country (originally 40 days) to prevent the spread of a disease within the country's borders. 3) The period of isolation following the onset of contagious disease. 4) The place where individuals are detained during a quarantine.

R

radiation therapy   The treatment of disease by radiation.

radiography   The making of film images (filming) of the internal structure of the body through exposure to x-radiation that acts on a sensitized film.

radioimmunoassay (RIA)   A highly sensitive method of determining the concentration of substances achieved by using the competition between radioactively labeled hormones and specific antibodies. It can be used to determine the concentration of: protein-bound hormones in blood plasma; any substance that causes the production of a specific antibody; or antibodies themselves.

radioimmunoprecipitation assay (RIPA)   A method of HIV antibody testing that is technically demanding and is used primarily in research. The virus is detected by the phenomenon of aggregation of sensitized antigen upon addition of specific antibody to antigen in solution (immunoprecipitation). The precipitate is then washed extensively, and disrupted and distributed through a polyacrylamide gel. Antibody-antigen bands are detected by autoradiography.

radiotherapy   The treatment of disease by the application of radiation.

receptive anal intercourse   Sexual intercourse in which an individual allows the insertion of a penis into his/her anus. This is a high-risk mode of transmission for the human immunodeficiency virus. *Also called* passive anal intercourse.

rectal douche   A current or stream of water directed against the rectum. It may be plain water or medicated.

133

rectal mucosa   A mucous membrane that lines the rectum.

rectum   The lower portion of the large intestine that is located between the sigmoid flexure and the anal canal.

red blood cell   *see* erythrocyte

red blood corpuscle   *see* erythrocyte

refractory   Recurring; not yielding to treatment.

Reiter's syndrome   A triad of symptoms consisting of arthritis, conjunctivitis, and urethritis, with urethritis generally appearing first but arthritis constituting the dominant feature. The syndrome is of unknown etiology and generally runs a self-limited but relapsing course.

remission   1) Abatement or diminution of the symptoms of a disease. 2) The period of time during which abatement or diminution of the symptoms of a disease occurs.

respirator   1) An apparatus or machine that can be used to artificially control ventilation. 2) A device that assists with pulmonary ventilation.

respiratory alkalosis   A metabolic condition resulting from an excessive loss of carbon dioxide from the lungs.

resuscitation   The restoration or revival of vital signs of life after apparent death.

reticuloendothelial cell   1) A phagocytic cell of the reticuloendothelial system. 2) A cell possessing the ability to isolate and ingest inert particles and vital dyes.

reticulosis   An abnormal increase in the number of cells related to reticuloendothelial cells.

retina   The innermost of three tunics of the eye. It receives images formed by the lens as light rays come to focus on the light-sensitive structure. The retina extends from the anterior entrance point of the optic nerve to the pupil. It is comprised of three parts: pars optica (the nervous or sensory portion that extends from the optic disk to the ora serrata, resting behind the ciliary process), pars ciliaris (the portion that lines the ciliary process), and pars iridica (the portion that rests on the posterior surface of the iris). The macula lutea, the most sensitive part of the retina, lies in the posterior portion of the retina. In the center of the macula lutea lies the depression called the fovea centralis. This is the region of most acute vision. Inside the fovea centralis is the point at which nerve fibers exit the retina to form the optic nerve. This point is called the optic papilla and is devoid of rods and cones, leaving it insensitive to light. From without, the retina is composed of pars pigmentosa (an outer pigment epithelium) and pars nervosa, which consists of nine layers (a layer of rods and cones, the external limiting membrane, the outer nuclear layer, the outer plexiform layer, the inner nuclear layer, the inner plexiform layer, the layer of ganglion cells, the nerve fiber layer, and the internal limiting membrane).

retinitis   Inflammation of the retina.

retinochoroiditis   *see* chorioretinitis

Retrovir   Past trade name of azidothymidine. The current trade name is Zidovudine.

retrovirus   The common name for the large family of RNA viruses that carry reverse transcriptase. These include the lentiviruses and leukoviruses.

rev gene   The gene in the human immunodeficiency virus that is required for viral protein RNA processing.

reverse transcriptase   Any enzyme that catalyzes the process of forming a compound by combining simpler molecules that synthesize DNA using certain aspects of RNA.

reverse transcriptase inhibitor   An agent that deters or prevents RNA-directed DNA polymerase. *See also* reverse transcriptase.

RIA   *see* radioimmunoassay

ribavirin   A synthetic nucleoside used as an antiviral.

ribonucleic acid (RNA)   A nucleic acid composed of ribonucleotide monomers. The base sequence of an RNA is dependent on the base sequence of a section of DNA that serves as a template for RNA synthesis (transcription). RNA controls protein synthesis in living cells and replaces DNA in certain viruses. *See also* deoxyribonucleic acid.

Rickettsia   A genus of bacteria made up of small, often multishaped microorganisms that are gram-negative and multiply only within the host cell. They are usually transmitted to humans by fleas, lice, mites, and ticks and are the causative agent of a variety of diseases including typhus fevers, spotted fevers, and scrub typhus.

Rifadin   *see* rifampin

rifampicin   *see* rifampin

rifampin   An antibiotic synthetically derived from rifamycin that appears as a red-brown, crystalline powder. It has the antibacterial properties of the rifamycin group and is used in the treatment of Mycobacterium tuberculosis. It is administered orally. *Also called* rifampicin. The trade names are Rimactane and Rifadin.

rifamycin   Any of a group of antibiotics biosynthesized by a strain of Streptomyces mediterranei and effective against a broad spectrum of bacteria, including gram-positive cocci, Mycobacterium tuberculosis, some gram-negative bacilli, and certain other mycobacteria.

Rimactane   *see* rifampin

rimming   *see* anilingus

ringworm   *see* tinea

RIPA   *see* radioimmunoprecipitation assay

risk group member   Any one of a group of individuals sharing common characteristics believed to place them at risk for infection with a communicable disease. (For example, people who have unprotected anal sex are at risk for infection with the human immunodeficiency virus.)

RNA   *see* ribonucleic acid

Robamox   *see* amoxicillin

route of transmission   The means by which a disease is passed or transferred from one individual to another.

Rubinstein, Arye   Born 1936 Tel Aviv, Israel, Rubinstein received his M.D. from the Medical Faculty, University of Bern, in 1962. He is currently a Professor at the Albert Einstein College of Medicine, Albert Einstein College Hospital in the Bronx, N.Y. Rubinstein was the first to describe immune deficiencies in children in the Bronx at the outset of the epidemic that were different from congenital immune problems. His work supported the theory that this immune deficiency was caused by a virus since it was being transmitted from mother to child, and that it was affecting groups beyond the homosexual community. Office address: 25 Astor Place, Monsey, NY 10952.

rush   *see* amyl nitrite inhalant and butyl nitrite inhalant

Ryan White CARE Bill   *see* Ryan White Comprehensive AIDS Resources Emergency Act of 1990.

Ryan White Comprehensive AIDS Resources Emergency Act of 1990 (CARE)   Legislation designed to direct relief to specific areas most affected by AIDS. The Act is divided into three sections: Title I, HIV Emergency Relief Grant program, provides emergency relief to HIV health care service programs in metropolitan areas with a cumulative total of more than 2,000 reported cases of AIDS; Title II, HIV CARE Grants, enables states to improve the quality, availability, and organization of care and support services in smaller cities and rural areas; Title III, Early Intervention Services, promotes early testing for HIV in order to prolong life and to modify behavior that endangers others at risk for infection.

Ryan White National Fund   Founded in 1986, this organization seeks to assist seriously ill children, particularly those with AIDS. It provides emergency financial aid, offers counseling, operates a referral service, promotes research, operates clinics, provides placement services, maintains a speakers' bureau, compiles statistics, and conducts education and awareness programs. The Fund is sponsored by Athletes and Entertainers for Kids, which is based at Nissan Motor Corporation, P.O. Box 191, Building B, Gardena, CA 90248-0191, (213) 276-5437.

S

S and M   *see* sadomasochism

sadism   1) The deriving of sexual pleasure from dominating, hurting, or mistreating one's partner. 2) The deriving of pleasure from inflicting physical or psychological pain on another or others. *See also* masochism.

sadomasochism (S and M)   1) Obtaining sexual pleasure from the practice of sadism or masochism. 2) Obtaining pleasure from the practice of sadism or masochism.

safe sex   The practice of protecting oneself and one's partner from viral transmission during sexual activities. Celibacy and masturbation are considered absolutely safe. The use of latex condoms is highly recommended for protection when engaging in sexual activities that could result in the exchange of body fluids. Use of the spermicide nonoxynol-9 is also recommended for added protection. Some authorities prefer the term safer sex, emphasizing that no form of sexual contact is 100 percent safe.

salivary-gland disease   A pathological condition involving the glands of the oral cavity that secrete saliva.

salivary gland virus   *see* cytomegalovirus

Salk, Jonas Edward   Born 1914 in New York City, Salk received his M.D. from New York University in 1939. Since 1975, he has served as the Founding Director of the Salk Institute of Biological Studies, and since 1984 as Distinguished Professor of International Health Sciences. Salk developed the poliovirus vaccine inactivated and has contributed to the research for a vaccine to prevent infection with the human immunodeficiency virus. Salk Institute of Biological Studies, P.O. Box 85800, San Diego, CA 92138.

Salk vaccine   *see* poliovirus vaccine inactivated

Salmonella   A genus of gram-negative bacteria belonging to the family Entobacteriaceae. Over 1,400 species have been identified, some of which are pathogenic. The most common manifestation is. food poisoning, ranging in severity from mild gastroenteritis to death.

salmonellosis   Any disease caused by infection with bacteria of the genus Salmonella. It can be manifested as gastroenteritis, septicemia, or typhoid fever.

San Francisco AIDS Foundation   Founded in 1982, this regional organization seeks to educate the public about HIV and AIDS prevention and provides various social services to people with the acquired immunodeficiency syndrome. The Foundation holds education workshops, forums, and seminars; disseminates educational materials and information; maintains a food bank and speakers' bureau; assists people with AIDS in obtaining emergency housing, government benefits, medical insurance, and legal referrals; conducts videotape training programs for health care providers and home health care workers to identify the needs of PWAs; produces various publications; and compiles statistics. Formerly called Kaposi's Sarcoma Research and Education Foundation. San Francisco AIDS Foundation, 333 Valencia Street, 4th Floor, San Francisco, CA 94103, (415) 864-4376.

Sandimmune   *see* cyclosporine A

sapphism   *see* lesbianism

scabies   A highly contagious dermatitis (skin inflammation) caused by Sarcoptes scabies, the itch mite. It is transmitted by close contact and is characterized by the eruption of papules, vesicles, and pustules. Eczema may result from scratching. *Also called* the itch and seven-year itch.

Schistosoma   1) A genus of parasites or flukes belonging to the family Schistosomatidae, class Trematoda, that thrive on blood. 2) The blood flukes.

schistosomiasis   A parasitic disease due to infestation with flukes of the genus Schistosoma.

SCID   *see* severe combined immunodeficiency

scrapie disease   One of the transmissible brain diseases in which the brain degenerates to the appearance of a sponge. It is characterized by severe itching, debility, and the inability to coordinate muscle movements. Scrapie disease generally occurs in sheep and goats and is inevitably fatal.

seborrhea   A functional disease of the sebaceous glands marked by the excessive secretion of sebum. *See also* seborrheic dermatitis.

seborrheic dermatitis   An acute or chronic inflammatory skin disease of unknown cause characterized by dry, moist, or greasy scaling and yellow or brown-gray crusted patches. It tends to especially involve the scalp but may include parts of the face, ears, genitalia, umbilicus, and supraorbital regions. *Also called* seborrhea and seborrheic eczema.

seborrheic eczema   *see* seborrheic dermatitis

semen   A thick, opalescent, whitish secretion of the male reproductive organs released at the climax of sexual excitement. Semen is the secretory product of various organs (prostate, bulbourethral glands, seminal vesicles, and others) plus spermatozoa. *Also called* sperm.

Sencer, David Judson   Born 1924 in Grand Rapids, Mich., Sencer received his M.D. from the University of Michigan in 1951 and his master's degree in public health from the Harvard School of Public Health in 1958. Since 1983, he has served as the Commissioner of the New York Health Department. Department of Community Medicine, Mount Sinai School of Medicine, 5th Avenue and 100th Street, New York, NY 10029.

Septra   *see* trimethoprim/sulfamethoxazole

seroconversion   The change of a test result from negative to positive, indicating the presence of antibodies in response to infection or vaccination.

Seromycin   *see* cycloserine

seronegative   Producing a negative result on serological tests; serologically negative; exhibiting no signs of antibody.

seropositive   Producing a positive result on serological tests; serologically positive; exhibiting definite signs of antibody.

seroprevalence   The number of individuals with evidence of antibodies against the causative agent of a disease in a given population at a specific period of time or at a particular point in time.

serostatus   The state or condition of a serologic test (i.e., seronegative or seropositive).

serum   1) The clear portion of any body fluid, especially that which moistens serous membranes. 2) The clear, watery portion of the blood that separates upon clotting. 3) Blood serum from an animal that has been immunized against a pathogenic organism that is used for passive immunization.

seven-year itch   *see* scabies

severe combined immunodeficiency (SCID)   A group of rare congenital disorders characterized by impairment of both humoral and cell-mediated immunity, manifested by lack of antibody formation in response to the presence of antigens, lack of delayed hypersensitivity, and inability to reject foreign tissue transplants. Without restoration of immune function or gnotobiotic isolation, death usually occurs by the first birthday as a result of opportunistic infection.

sex club   Any of a group of facilities dedicated to the promotion of the pursuit of sexual pleasure (e.g., bathhouses, orgy rooms).

sexual intercourse   Sexual activity involving genital contact between individuals. Some definitions confine sexual intercourse to the joining of the sexual organs of a male and a female human being, in which the erect penis is inserted into the vagina, usually with the ejaculation of semen into the vagina. *See also* anal intercourse, vaginal intercourse.

sexually transmitted disease (STD)   Disease acquired as a result of sexual contact (heterosexual or homosexual) with an infected partner. This term is more inclusive than venereal disease, since it includes certain conditions that can also be acquired by nonsexual means (e.g., amebiasis or shigellosis).

Sezary syndrome   1) A skin disease characterized by shedding. 2) A form of cutaneous T-cell lymphoma characterized by exfoliative dermatitis, severe itching, peripheral lymphadenopathy, and abnormal hyperchromatic mononuclear cells in the lymph nodes, skin, and peripheral blood.

Shanti Project   Founded in 1975, this organization is divided into regional groups that provide volunteer counseling services to people who are affected by the acquired immunodeficiency syndrome or the human immunodeficiency virus. Volunteers are matched with clients based on a variety of identified needs in the belief that peer counseling can help people achieve the inner peace necessary to confront fears, frustration, isolation, depression, sorrow, and stress. The project also educates health care workers and laypersons, produces various publications, organizes support groups, provides practical assistance, and offers long-term, low-cost housing to eligible people with AIDS. Shanti Project, 525 Howard Street, San Francisco, CA 94105, (415) 777-CARE.

Shigella   A genus of gram-negative, non-motile, rod-shaped bacteria of the family Enterobacteriaceae that ferment carbohydrates with acid but do not produce gas. The genus consists of several species, all of which normally inhabit the intestinal tract of humans and cause digestive disturbances ranging from diarrhea to severe dysentery.

shigellosis   The disease produced by organisms of the genus Shigella.

shingles   1) The nontechnical name for herpes zoster. 2) The eruption of acute, inflammatory, herpetic vesicles along the area of the affected nerve. The disease represents reactivation of varicella zoster virus (chickenpox). *See also* herpes zoster.

shooting gallery   A facility established for the explicit use of the illegal sale and abuse of intravenous drugs.

sickle cell anemia   1) An inherited chronic anemia characterized by an abnormal red blood cell that contains a defective form of hemoglobin causing the cell to become sickle-shaped when deprived of oxygen. 2) An inherited anemia characterized by the presence of crescent-shaped (sickle-shaped) erythrocytes and by accelerated hemolysis.

sickle cell disease   *see* sickle cell anemia

sigmoidoscope   A flexible or rigid instrument used to examine the lower colon (sigmoid flexure).

sigmoidoscopy   Inspection of the sigmoid colon (the lower portion of the descending colon, located between the iliac crest and the rectum, which is shaped like the letter S) using a sigmoidoscope.

sign   Any objective evidence discoverable upon examination of a patient, indicative of disease. *See also* symptom.

Silverman, Mervyn F.   Born 1938 in Washington, D.C., Silverman received his M.D. from Tulane University in 1964. He is currently a Medical Administrator and Adjunct Professor at the University of California, San Francisco. Silverman was Director of the San Francisco Department of Public Health at the outset of the epidemic. Office address: 119 Frederick Street, San Francisco, CA 94117.

simian immunodeficiency virus (SIV)   Any of a group of viruses structurally similar to the human immunodeficiency virus found in monkeys. *Also called* simian T-lymphotrophic virus (STLV).

simian retrovirus   Any of a group of retroviruses found in monkeys.

simian T-lymphotrophic virus (STLV)   *see* simian immunodeficiency virus

sinusitis   Inflammation of a sinus.

SIV   *see* simian immunodeficiency virus

slim disease   *see* HIV wasting syndrome

Social Security Administration   Established by Reorganization Plan No. 2 of 1946, the Administration oversees a national program of contributory social insurance whereby employees, employers, and the self-employed pay contributions that are pooled in special trust funds. The United States is divided into ten regions, each headed by a Regional Commissioner. Each region contains a network of district offices, branch offices, and teleservice centers, which serve as the contact points between the Administration and the public. These installations are responsible for informing people of the purposes and provisions of programs and their rights and responsibilities thereunder; assisting with claims filed for retirement, survivors, health, or disability insurance benefits, black lung benefits, or supplemental security income; developing and adjudicating claims; assisting certain beneficiaries in claiming reimbursement for medical expenses; conducting development of cases involving earnings records, coverage, and fraud-related questions; making rehabilitation service referrals; and assisting claimants in filing appeals on Administration determination of benefit entitlements or amounts. Office of Public Inquiries, Social Security Administration, Department of Health and Human Services, 6401 Security Boulevard, Baltimore, MD 21235, (301) 965-7700.

sonography   *see* ultrasonography

Southern blot technique   A procedure used to separate and identify DNA sequences in which DNA fragments are separated by electrophoresis onto an agarose gel, blotted onto a nylon or nitrocellulose membrane, and hybridized with labeled nucleic acid probes.

sperm   1) The semen or testicular secretion, containing spermatozoa, ejaculated from the male. 2) Spermatozoa.

spermatozoa   Plural of spermatozoon.

spermatozoon   The mature male germ cell that is formed within the seminiferous tubules of the testes. It consists of a head with a nucleus, a neck, a middle piece, and a tail and resembles a tadpole in shape. Spermatozoon is the element of semen concerned with reproduction that pierces the envelope of the ovum to achieve fertilization.

spermicide   An agent that destroys spermatozoa.

spiramycin   An antibiotic produced from a member of the Streptomyces bacteria. It is administered orally.

splenic fever   *see* anthrax

splenomegaly   Enlargement of the spleen.

Sporothrix schenckii   A species of the genus Sporothrix, a di-
morphic imperfect fungi that is the causative agent of sporotrichosis.
It grows in soil or vegetation (especially in thorny bushes) and is
transmitted when infected thorns enter subcutaneous tissues. It also
grows as a yeast and parasitizes tissue as a yeast at 37°C.

sporotrichosis   A chronic fungal infection caused by Sporothrix
schenckii that is characterized by abscesses, nodules, and ulcers of
the skin and adjacent lymph nodes. The infection may remain localized, or it may spread throughout the body via the bloodstream.

sprue   A disease characterized by weakness, weight loss, anemia,
and malabsorption of essential elements. It occurs in both tropical
and nontropical forms. The cause is unknown.

sputum   Matter ejected from the bronchi, lungs, and trachea through
the mouth.

sputum examination   The microscopic inspection of expectorated
matter (especially mucus or mucopurulent matter ejected in diseases
involving the air passages) for the purpose of diagnosis.

squamous cell   A flat, scalelike, epithelial cell.

squamous cell carcinoma   A carcinoma developing from squamous
epithelium.

Staphylococcus   A genus of aerobic to facultatively anaerobic,
nonmotile, non-spore-forming bacteria containing gram-positive,
spherical cells that divide in multiple planes to form irregular clus-
ters resembling grapes. Under anaerobic conditions, they produce
lactic acid from glucose; under aerobic conditions, they produce acetic
acid and small amounts of carbon dioxide. Certain strains (coagulase-
positive) produce various toxins that are potentially pathogenic and
may cause food poisoning. They are found on the skin, skin glands,
mucous and nasal membranes, as well as in various food products.

Staphylococcus aureus   A species of Staphylococcus commonly
found on the skin and mucous membranes, especially those of the
mouth and nose. They are characterized by the production of golden-
yellow pigment and are gram-positive and coagulase positive. They

cause serious suppurative conditions and systemic diseases. Various strains of the species produce toxins that cause food poisoning and toxic shock syndrome.

STD *see* sexually transmitted disease

sterilization 1) The destruction of all microorganisms in, on, or about an object by employing various means such as chemical agents (alcohol, ethylene oxide gas, phenol), high-velocity electron bombardment, steam, or ultraviolet light radiation. 2) The act or process by which an individual is made incapable of reproduction or fertilization (e.g., castration, tubectomy, vasectomy).

Stevens-Johnson syndrome A form of erythema multiforme (eruption of dark red papules or tubercles) that is sometimes fatal. It is characterized by systemic exfoliative mucocutaneous lesions, some of which may be severe. The lesions may involve the ears, nose, lips, eyes, anus, genitals, lungs, gastrointestinal tract, heart, and kidneys.

stigma 1) A mark of disgrace or reproach. 2) Something that detracts from the character of a person or group.

STLV *see* simian immunodeficiency virus

stomatitis Inflammation of the mouth.

straight *see* heterosexual

streptomycin A bacterial antibiotic derived from the soil microbe Streptomyces griseus. It belongs to the aminoglycoside class and is effective against most gram-negative and acid-fast bacteria. It is also effective against certain gram-positive forms but is used mainly in the treatment of tuberculosis.

stroke A condition characterized by paralysis and often some irreversible neurologic damage. It can include focal weakness, speech impediment, and impaired consciousness and is caused by acute vascular lesions of the brain such as hemorrhage, embolism, or thrombosis. *Also called* cerebrovascular accident and stroke syndrome.

stroke syndrome *see* stroke

Strongyloides stercoralis   A roundworm occurring in tropical and subtropical countries and in the Southern U.S. that infects dogs, primates, and humans. The female and larvae inhabit the intestines of the host, where they cause diarrhea and ulceration. The rod-shaped larvae are expelled in the stool and may pass through the venous system to the lungs, where they cause hemorrhage (pulmonary strongyloidiasis). From the lungs they migrate upwards and reach the intestines via the trachea and esophagus. Infestation may persist for years due to the nature of the life cycle. Massive infections may be seen in patients treated with immunosuppressive drugs or in immunosuppressed states. Infection may be fatal.

strongyloidiasis   Infection with nematodes of the genus Strongyloides. Infection can occur indirectly by larvae of a new generation developed in the soil; directly by infective larvae developed without an intervening adult phase; or by autoreinfection, where larvae develop within the intestinal feces of the host, penetrate the mucosa, and migrate back to the intestines through blood-lung interactions. Autoreinfection is the cause of most serious human infections and the majority of fatalities. *Also called* strongyloidosis. *See also* Strongyloides stercoralis.

strongyloidosis   *see* strongyloidiasis

subacute encephalitis   *see* AIDS dementia complex

sulfadiazine   A derivative of sulfonamide that appears as a white or yellowish powder. Because of its ability to penetrate the blood-brain barrier, it is used in the treatment of some types of meningitis. Sulfadiazine is also used to treat infections involving susceptible organisms such as acute urinary tract infections and chancroid. It is administered orally.

sulfamethoxazole   A sulfonamide appearing as a white to off-white crystalline powder that is used in the treatment of urinary tract infections. It is administered orally.

sulfonamide   Any of a group of compounds that consist of the amides of sulfamic acid. They are derivatives of sulfanilamide and are bacteriostatic. Their action on bacteria results from their ability to interfere with the functioning of the enzyme systems required for normal metabolism, growth, and multiplication.

Supplementary Security Income (SSI)   A basic federal payment program administered by the Social Security Administration for the aged, blind, and disabled. It is financed out of general revenue. *See also* Social Security Administration.

support group   A group whose purpose is to give courage, confidence, or faith to each other. Most often associated with psychotherapy. *See also* support network.

support network   A group of interconnected or cooperative individuals who give courage, confidence, or faith to each other. A support network tends to be less formal in nature than a support group (e.g., family or friends).

suppressor cell   A subset of T lymphocytes that inhibits B lymphocyte antibody formation and is involved in autoimmunity and immune tolerance. *See also* lymphocyte.

suppurative   Forming pus.

suramin   The first compound identified in 1984 with anti-HIV activity in vitro, it entered clinical trials for patients with Kaposi's sarcoma and AIDS-related complex. The drug was found to be highly toxic, with no clinical, immunologic, or virologic benefit to HIV-infected individuals.

surgeon general   The chief medical officer in the U.S. Army, Air Force, Navy, or Public Health Service.

surveillance   1) The monitoring, watching, or controlling of something. 2) The procedure of closely monitoring the contacts of individuals exposed to an infectious disease during the incubation period to prevent the spread of the disease. Surveillance is sometimes used in place of quarantine. *See also* quarantine.

susceptible host   Any organism that is easily invaded by a parasitic organism for the purpose of subsistence, especially for nourishment.

symptom   1) Any perceptive change in the body or bodily functions indicative of disease, kinds of disease, or phases of disease. They may be classed as objective, subjective, cardinal, and constitutional; however, all symptoms are generally classed as subjective, with objective indications being considered signs. 2) Any change in a patient's condition indicative of mental or physical illness.

synergy   Action of two or more agents or drugs working together; cooperation.

synthetic baryta   *see* barium sulfate

syphilis   A subacute to chronic, infectious, venereal disease characterized by lesions that may involve any organ or body tissue. Generally, cutaneous manifestations are exhibited, and relapses may occur frequently. Syphilis may remain asymptomatic for years. It is usually transmitted through sexual contact (both heterosexual and homosexual), but may be acquired in utero or by direct contact with infected tissue or blood. If untreated, syphilis progresses through three clinical stages: primary (initial painless ulceration lesions at the site of inoculation); secondary (widespread mucocutaneous lesions and generalized regional lymphadenopathy); and tertiary (destructive lesions involving many organs and tissues, including the heart and central nervous system).

systemic   1) Relating to the entire organism as distinguished from any of its individual parts. 2) Relating to a system.

systemic disease   Any pathologic condition involving the entire organism as opposed to an individual organ system or part.

T

T cell   *see* T lymphocyte

T-cell count   Calculation of the number of T lymphocytes in a cubic millimeter of blood.

T-cell leukemia   *see* T-cell lymphoma

T-cell lymphoma   An acute or subacute disease associated with a human T-cell virus and characterized by lymphadenopathy, hypercalcemia, hepatosplenomegaly, skin lesions, and peripheral blood involvement. *Also called* T-cell leukemia.

T-cell ratio   The ratio of T4 lymphocytes (helper cells) to T8 lymphocytes (suppressor cells) in the blood.

T4 cells   Helper cells that assist in the production of antibody-forming cells from B lymphocytes. *See also* T lymphocyte.

T lymphocyte   A thymocyte-derived lymphocyte that is long-lived and of immunological importance, since it is responsible for cell-mediated immunity. *Also called* T cell.

T lymphocyte, helper cell   CD4 lymphocyte. *See also* helper cell and lymphocyte.

T lymphocyte, suppressor cell   CD8 lymphocyte. *See also* suppressor cell and lymphocyte.

tat gene   The gene that encodes a transactivating genetic element of the human immunodeficiency virus that increases the production of cellular and viral proteins.

Teens Teaching AIDS Prevention   Founded in 1987, this organization seeks to inform teenagers about HIV and AIDS through peer education. It operates a toll-free hotline staffed by trained teenagers with adult advisers, maintains a speakers' bureau, and provides companions for youths with AIDS. Teens Teaching AIDS Prevention, 3030 Walnut, Kansas City, MO 64108, (816) 561-8784, (800) 234-TEEN (hotline).

terminal-stage   Pertaining to the end phase.

testicular atrophy   A wasting away, or decrease in size and function, of the testis (male reproductive gland located in the cavity of the scrotum).

testicular carcinoma   A malignant neoplasm occurring in the male reproductive gland (testis).

testing   1) The procedure used to determine the presence or nature of a substance or disease. 2) Producing a significant chemical reaction.

tetracycline   Any of a group of broad-spectrum antibiotics belonging to certain species of Streptomyces. They may also be produced semisynthetically. The tetracyclines are effective against a variety of organisms, including gram-negative and gram-positive bacteria, chlamydias, mycoplasmas, rickettsias, and some viruses and protozoa. Trade names are Tetracyn and SK-Tetracycline.

Tetracyn   *see* tetracycline

therapy   The treatment of a disease or pathological condition. *See also* treatment.

thrombocytopenia   A condition in which there is a decrease in the number of platelets in circulating blood. *Also called* thrombopenia.

thrombopenia   *see* thrombocytopenia

thrush   *see* oral candidiasis

thymidine   1) A nucleoside that is one of the basic components of deoxyribonucleic acid (DNA). 2) A nucleoside present in deoxyribonucleotide.

TIA   *see* transient ischemic attack

Tinactin   *see* tolnaftate

tinea   Any fungus skin disease involving various parts of the body, with the specific type indicating the part involved. (Tinea barbae affects the beard.) *Also called* ringworm.

TMP/SMX   *see* trimethoprim/sulfamethoxazole

tolnaftate   A synthetic antifungal agent appearing as a white to creamy white powder. It is used topically in treating various forms of tinea. The trade name is Tinactin.

toot   *see* cocaine

topical   Pertaining to a specific surface area.

torulosis   *see* cryptococcosis

toxic shock syndrome (TSS)   A rare disease caused by toxins that are produced by certain strains of Staphylococcus aureus bacteria. It is characterized by acute high fever, diarrhea, vomiting, and myalgia (tenderness or pain in the muscles), followed by hypotension and possible death due to shock. It mostly affects young menstruating women using tampons, but cases also have been diagnosed in non-menstruating women, as well as in males.

toxicity   The quality of being poisonous.

Toxoplasma gondii   An intracellular, non-host-specific, widespread, sporozoan species that is parasitic in a variety of vertebrates, including humans. The sexual cycle, leading to the production of oocysts, develops exclusively in cats and other felines. Infection from ingestion of oocysts, tissue cysts in raw meat, or transplacental migration allows the proliferative stages and tissue cysts to develop in a variety of animal species in utero. It is the causative agent of toxoplasmosis.

toxoplasmosis   An acute or chronic disease caused by infection with the protozoa Toxoplasma gondii. The organism is found in many mammals and birds, but the definitive host is the feces of cats. In humans, infection is usually asymptomatic. When symptoms do appear, they may range from a mild, self-limited disease similar to mononucleosis to a more severe, disseminated disease (encephalitis, hepatitis, or pneumonitis) causing extensive damage to the brain, central nervous system, liver, and lungs. The immunocompromised patient and transplacentally infected fetus are the most susceptible to severe manifestations.

transfusion   The injection of whole blood or a blood component into the bloodstream.

transfusion-associated AIDS   The development of the acquired immunodeficiency syndrome as a result of a transfusion with HIV-infected blood or blood components. Most experts believe that the risk of becoming infected with HIV through a blood transfusion is now remote because of widespread, accurate blood-testing procedures.

transient ischemic attack (TIA)   The temporary interruption of the blood supply to the brain. The symptoms and signs of neurologic deficit may last from a few minutes to hours but are not persistent. No evidence of residual brain damage or neurologic damage exists after the attack.

transmission   1) The conveyance of disease from one individual to another. 2) The passage of a nerve impulse across a synapse. 3) Transfer.

Treponema pallidum   The causative agent of syphilis in humans.

triage   The sorting out and classifying of sick, injured, or wounded persons. This term was developed during wartime and is used in times of disaster. Triage determines the priority of medical need of patients and assigns placement for treatment in order of severity, life-threatening nature, and survival potential. It provides a way to promote efficient use of health care personnel, facilities, and equipment to the maximum benefit of all patients.

trial accrual   The number of persons enrolled in a clinical trial at a given time.

Trichomonas hominis   *see* Pentatrichomonas hominis

Trichomonas vaginalis   A species of parasitic protozoan flagellates, belonging to the genus Trichomonas, that are commonly found in the urethra and vagina of women and in the urethra and prostate gland of men. It is the causative agent of trichomoniasis vaginitis.

trichomoniasis vaginitis   Acute or subacute urethritis or vaginitis due to infection with Trichomonas vaginalis that does not invade the tissue or mucosa but causes an inflammatory reaction. Infection is venereal or by other forms of contact. It is usually asymptomatic but may produce vaginitis, with vulvar and vaginal pruritus, vaginal discharge of white or yellowish viscid fluid containing mucus and pus, and rarely purulent urethritis in males.

trimethoprim   An antimicrobial agent that enhances the effect of sulfonamides and sulfones.

trimethoprim/sulfamethoxazole (TMP/SMX)   A drug combination of trimethoprim and sulfamethoxazole that is used in the treatment of Pneumocystis carinii pneumonia and infection with Isospora belli. Trade names are Bactrim and Septra.

trimetrexate   An antineoplastic agent and antiprotozoal orphan drug used in the treatment of Pneumocystis carinii pneumonia.

Trimox   *see* amoxicillin

trip   A vernacular term used to denote a drug-induced period of hallucination or euphoria.

TSS   *see* toxic shock syndrome

tubercle   1) A granulomatous lesion caused by infection with Mycobacterium tuberculosis. They vary in size and in histologic component proportions but tend to be circumscribed, firm, spheroidal lesions that generally consist of three zones: an inner focus of necrosis; a middle zone, consisting of an accumulation of large mononuclear phagocytes, or macrophages (Langhans type multinucleated giant cells may also be present); and an outer zone, consisting mostly of numerous lymphocytes with a few monocytes and plasma cells. Where healing has begun, fibrous tissue forming at the periphery may form a fourth zone. 2) A term used nonspecifically to refer to granuloma.

tuberculosis   Any infectious disease caused by the Mycobacterium, with the most common causative agent being Mycobacterium tuberculosis. It is characterized by inflammatory infiltrations, formation of tubercles, caseous necrosis, abscesses, calcification, and fibrosis. Tuberculosis most commonly affects the respiratory system but may affect other parts of the body such as the gastrointestinal tract, bones, and skin. Infection is usually through contact with an infected person or animal.

typhoid fever   1) An acute infectious disease acquired by ingesting food or water contaminated by waste matter excreted from the body, characterized by fever. 2) An acute infectious disease characterized by sustained bacteremia and infestation of the pathogen within the mononuclear phagocytic cells of the liver, lymph nodes, spleen, and Peyer's patches of the ileum, accompanied by fever, rash, headache, malaise, and abdominal pain. Diagnosis is made by isolation of the bacteria from the blood.

typhus   An acute infectious disease caused by rickettsiae and occurring in two forms: endemic typhus (murine) and epidemic typhus (louse-bourne).

U

ulcer   A local defect, lesion, or open sore of the skin or mucous membrane that is accompanied by the sloughing of inflammatory necrotic (dead or decaying) tissue. Pus may be discharged if the sore becomes infected.

ulceration   1) The development or formation of an ulcer. 2) An ulcer.

ultrasonic cardiography   *see* echocardiography

ultrasonography   The use of ultrasonic waves to visualize or photograph an organ or tissue by recording the echoes or pulses of the waves as they are projected from the tissues.

uremia   1) An excessive amount of nitrogenous substances (e.g., urea or creatinine) in the blood that are normally excreted by the kidney. 2) The constellation of symptoms associated with the toxic condition caused by chronic or acute renal failure, including anorexia, nausea, and vomiting. *See also* azotemia.

urethritis   Inflammation of the urethra.

V

vaccination The introduction of any vaccine into the body to establish resistance to a specific infectious disease. *See also* immunization.

vaccine The incorporation of weakened or killed microorganisms with a suitable liquid for administration in order to prevent or treat an infectious disease.

vacuolar myelopathy A pathologic condition involving vacuolization (the formation of vacuoles) and sometimes degeneration of the spinal cord.

vacuole 1) A clear place in the substance of a cell. Sometimes it is degenerative in character; sometimes it surrounds a foreign body and serves as a temporary stomach for digestion of that foreign matter. 2) A minute space found in any tissue.

vaginal intercourse Sexual intercourse by insertion of the penis into the vagina.

vaginal secretion 1) The substance produced by glands in the vagina. 2) The process whereby cells of the glands in the vagina produce materials from the blood.

vaginitis Inflammation of the vagina.

varicella-zoster virus A herpetovirus that causes herpes zoster and varicella (chickenpox) in humans. Herpes zoster results from secondary infection by varicella-zoster virus or by reactivation of infection that may have been latent for some years. Varicella results from primary infection with varicella-zoster virus.

vasopressin   1) A hormone formed by the neuronal cells of the hypothalamic nuclei and transported to the posterior lobe of the hypophysis (pituitary gland), where it is stored through the hypothalamohypophyseal tract. It stimulates the contraction of the muscular tissue of the capillaries and arterioles, elevating blood pressure. 2) A pharmaceutical preparation of similar nature, extracted from the posterior pituitary of domestic animals or produced synthetically. It is used as an antidiuretic in the treatment of acute or chronic diabetes insipidus. *Also called* antidiuretic hormone. The trade name is Pitressin.

VD   *see* venereal disease

venereal disease (VD)   Any pathologic condition acquired through sexual intercourse (heterosexual or homosexual) with an infected partner. *See also* sexually transmitted disease.

venereal wart   *see* condyloma acuminatum

Veterans Benefits Administration   The Administration conducts an integrated program of veterans benefits including compensation and pension, vocational rehabilitation and education, loan guaranties, and other forms of veteran assistance. It is one of three organizations that constitute the Department of Veterans Affairs and has a central office as well as field facilities. Public Affairs Officer, Veterans Benefits Administration, Department of Veterans Affairs, 810 Vermont Avenue, N.W., Washington, DC 20420, (202) 233-5210.

vidarabine   An antiviral agent that inhibits DNA synthesis and is effective in the treatment of herpes simplex and herpes zoster-varicella viruses. It has also been show to be effective against herpes simplex encephalitis. *Also called* adenine arabinoside and ara-A. The trade name is Vira-A.

Videx   *see* dideoxyinosine

vif gene   The gene in the human immunodeficiency virus that encodes proteins of 23,000 molecular weight and effects virus replication by increasing virus production.

villoma   *see* papilloma

villous papilloma   *see* papilloma

villous tumor   *see* papilloma

vinblastine sulfate   1) A drug that prevents the development, growth, or proliferation of malignant cells. 2) An antineoplastic drug obtained from Vinca rosea used in the treatment of Hodgkin's disease, Kaposi's sarcoma, choriocarcinoma, acute and chronic leukemias, and other neoplastic disorders. *See also* vincristine sulfate.

vincristine sulfate   1) A drug that prevents the development, growth, or proliferation of malignant cells. 2) An antineoplastic drug obtained from Vinca rosea with similar activity to vinblastine, but more useful in the treatment of acute leukemia and lymphocytic lymphosarcoma.

Vira-A   *see* vidarabine

viral encephalitis   Encephalitis caused by a virus.

virology   The study of viruses and viral diseases.

virus   A minute infectious organism not visible under an ordinary light microscope. These organisms are, however, visible in electron microscopy and are characterized by their entire dependency upon host cells for their metabolic and reproductive needs. They consist of nucleic acid, a strand of DNA or RNA (but not both), and a protein covering. Viruses may be classified according to the host they dominate: bacteria, animal, or plant. They are also classed according to their origin, mode of transmission, manifestation they produce in the host, and geographic location where they are first isolated.

Visiting Nurse Associations of America   Founded in 1983, this organization consists of voluntary, nonprofit, home health care agencies. It seeks to develop competitive strength among its members, develop business resources, institute economic programs, issue public service announcements, produce various publications, and conduct workshops and training seminars. Visiting Nurse Associations of America, 1391 N. Speer Boulevard, #802, P.O. Box 4637, Denver, CO 80204, (303) 629-8622.

visna   A viral disease that affects sheep. The primary target is the central nervous system. It is characterized by asymptomatic onset and partial paralysis of the hind limbs, progressing to total paralysis and death.

vitamin M   *see* folic acid

Volberding, Paul Arthur   Born 1949, Volberding received his M.D. from the University of Minnesota. He is currently a member of the Department of Hematology, University of California, San Francisco. Volberding was one of the first to work with Kaposi's sarcoma patients in San Francisco at the outset of the pandemic. Department of Hematology, Medical Center, University of California, San Francisco, CA 94143.

von Willebrand's disease   A congenital bleeding disorder. It usually manifests at an early age, with the symptoms decreasing with age or during pregnancy. It is characterized by prolonged periods of bleeding and a deficient amount of coagulation Factor VIII in the blood. It is associated with increased bleeding during surgery or trauma and excessive loss of blood during menstruation.

vpr gene   The gene in the human immunodeficiency virus whose function is presently unknown.

vulvovaginal condition   The state of health pertaining to the vulva and vagina.

W

wart A circumscribed elevation of the skin resulting from an increase in size or bulk of the epidermis and protuberances in the layer just under the epidermis. Warts are caused by a papillomavirus.

wasting syndrome *see* HIV wasting syndrome

water sport Sexual activity involving urination. *See also* golden shower.

Watkins Commission *see* Presidential Commission on the Human Immunodeficiency Virus Epidemic

Watkins, James D. Chairman of Ronald Reagan's Presidential Commission on the Human Immunodeficiency Virus Epidemic (better known as the Watkins Commission). The Commission supported the creation of a national registry of clinical trials for all AIDS drugs in 1988, increasing access to trials.

Western blot 1) A blood test used to detect antibodies to HIV and to confirm ELISA test results. 2) A test used for analyzing protein antigens. Antigens are separated by changing the electrical potential (electrophoresis) and are then transferred to a solid substance by blotting. The substance or membrane is incubated with antibodies. Enzymatic or radioactive techniques are then used to detect the bound antibodies. This method is very precise and is used for detecting small quantities of antibodies.

Whipple's disease A malabsorption syndrome characterized by abnormal skin pigmentation, diarrhea, weight loss, weakness, arthritis, lymphadenopathy, and lesions of the central nervous system.

WHO *see* World Health Organization

will   1) A legal statement of an individual's wishes concerning the disposal of his/her property after death. 2) The mental capacity for making a reasoned choice or decision. 3) The strength and power of controlling one's own actions.

works   Slang term for paraphernalia used by substance abusers for the illicit intravenous injection of drugs.

World Health Organization (WHO)   Founded in 1948, this international organization is the health agency of the United Nations. Its goal is to achieve the optimum level of health care for all people. Objectives of the WHO include directing and coordinating international health work, ensuring technical cooperation, promoting research, preventing and controlling disease, and generating and disseminating information. The Organization emphasizes and supports the health needs of developing countries; establishes standards for biological, food, and pharmaceutical needs; and determines environmental health criteria. World Health Organization, Avenue Appia, CH-1211 Geneva 27, Switzerland, 22 7912111.

World Health Organization Collaborating Centre on AIDS   Founded in 1985, this health agency is chartered by the World Health Organization to conduct research and education and training programs concerning HIV and AIDS in order to promote public health. World Health Organization Collaborating Centre on AIDS, c/o Centers for Disease Control and Prevention, 1600 Clifton Road, N.E., Atlanta, GA 30333, (404) 639-3311.

World Hemophilia AIDS Center   Founded in 1984, this organization functions as a clearinghouse for information concerning AIDS and hemophilia patients. The Center also collects data and conducts research to determine the extent of infection among hemophiliacs. World Hemophilia AIDS Center, 10 Congress Street, Suite 340, Pasadena, CA 91105, (818) 577-4366.

X, Y, Z

xerosis   Abnormal dryness of the skin, mouth, or eyes.

Yarchoan, Robert   Born 1950 in New York City, Yarchoan received his M.D. from the University of Pennsylvania in 1975. He is currently an Academic Senior Investigator for the National Cancer Institute. Yarchoan has worked on several possible drug therapies for AIDS. National Institutes of Health Clinical Center, NIH Building 10, 12N248, Bethesda, MD 20892, (301) 496-5387.

yeast   A general term including any of several unicellular, usually rounded fungi that reproduce by budding. Some transform to a mold stage under certain environmental conditions, while others remain unicellular. A few yeasts are pathogenic in humans.

yeast infection   Invasion and multiplication of yeasts in body tissues that may produce injurious effects.

yellow nail syndrome   A syndrome associated with an excessive amount of tissue fluids in the body tissues due to obstruction of the lymphatics, especially of the legs. The nails become yellowish to greenish in color and may be smooth, thickened, or excessively curved, slow in growth, and loose, causing them to be shed.

Yodoxin   *see* iodoquinol

Zidovudine   *see* azidothymidine

zoophilic sexual contact   Preference for sexual contact with animals rather than humans.

FOR MORE INFORMATION

For more information, contact the National AIDS Hotline at 1-800-342-2437, the National AIDS Clearinghouse at 1-800-458-5231, or your local AIDS service provider.

Dr. Jeffrey Huber is currently an Assistant Professor at the School of Library and Information Studies, Texas Woman's University. He received his Ph.D. in Library Science, specializing in HIV/AIDS information, from the University of Pittsburgh.